Colitis

Ulcerative colitis, a chronic condition with many long-term complications, also poses certain short-term problems for the sufferer. In *Colitis*, the latest title in The Experience of Illness series, Michael Kelly considers the reality of living and coping with a condition that is constantly unpredictable, generally debilitating and presents the threat of a long-term major decline in health.

He outlines and assesses the curative surgery that is sometimes performed, namely total colectomy and ileostomy, and discusses the various strategies which sufferers develop and adopt in order to keep their condition under control.

Of immense value to all health professionals who care for and counsel people with colitis, the book will also provide help and encouragement to sufferers, their families and friends.

Michael Kelly is Senior Lecturer in the Department of Public Health at Glasgow University.

The Experience of Illness

Series Editors: Ray Fitzpatrick and Stanton Newman

Colitis

Michael P. Kelly

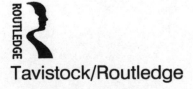

Tavistock/Routledge

First published in 1992
by Routledge
11 New Fetter Lane, London EC4P 4EE

Simultaneously published in the USA and Canada
by Routledge
a division of Routledge, Chapman and Hall Inc.
29 West 35th Street, New York, NY10001

© 1992 Michael P. Kelly

Typeset in Times by
NWL Editorial Services, Langport, Somerset

Printed and bound in Great Britain by
Mackays of Chatham PLC, Chatham, Kent

British Library Cataloguing in Publication Data
A catalogue record for this book is available from
the British Library

Library of Congress Cataloging in Publication Data
Kelly, Michael P.
    Colitis / Michael P. Kelly.
    p.   cm. (The Experience of Illness)
    Includes bibliographical references and index.
    1. Ulcerative colitis. 2. Ileostomy. I. Title. II. Series.
    [DNLM: 1. Colitis, Ulcerative – psychology.   2. Colitis,
    Ulcerative – surgery.   WI 522 K285c]
    RC862.C63K45   1992
    616.3'447 – dc20
    DNLM/DLC for Library of Congress

ISBN 0–415–03839–1

Contents

Preface

This is a book about the experiences of men and women who have had ulcerative colitis and have had that disease cured surgically. The main subject matter is the words of people describing their experiences. The book tries to provide an authentic representation of what it is like to be ill with colitis, to undergo major surgery, and to live with an ileostomy. The idea which is implicit or explicit in most patients' and ex patients' descriptions of their experiences is 'coping'. They talk about how they coped with their symptoms, their pain, their distress and their recovery. The central sociological and psychological organizing concept in the text is therefore coping.

The main audience for this text will probably be professionals with an interest, such as doctors, nurses or stoma therapists, in colitis and its sequelae. A sub-theme in the book is to show what the disciplines of sociology and psychology can contribute to an understanding of the patient's experience and can contribute to the care of such patients. The book may also be of interest to medical sociologists and medical psychologists as an example of the application of aspects of their disciplines to a specific disease. I hope too that the book will be of interest to lay readers. Patients and relatives may find some comfort in the text. This is not because the book contains a message of hope (there are no miracle cures or strange psychological theories here) but rather because the realization that someone with colitis is not suffering alone may be helpful. One of the very surprising things about doing the research for this book was the discovery that many people with colitis had never spoken to anyone, other than their doctor and close relatives, about their illness and that they had little conception of a group of other people in a similar predicament until after they had surgery. To the lay reader who has the disease or to the relative of a sufferer, there may be some consolation in the sharing of experience.

My qualifications for writing this book are twofold. First, I am a sociologist with a smattering of psychology, and on that basis I researched the experiences of people with colitis in the Department of Psychiatry at the University of Dundee. Second, I contracted ulcerative colitis long before I became a sociologist. I had the disease for nineteen years and it was eventually cured when I was 30 by the surgical removal of my colon, anus and rectum. I now have an ileostomy. The experience of colitis and colectomy is therefore something with which I, and my family, are very familiar. Inevitably this book reflects my personal experiences, but overlaid, I hope, by my scientific training.

Michael P. Kelly, 1992

Acknowledgements

In preparing this book very many people have helped, advised or supported me. My wife Tessa has endured the inconvenience of a husband who periodically needed to write, or be engaged in research, when time could, or should have been spent together. Likewise our children, Paul, Rachel and Helen, have had to put up with mounds of paper and books in various rooms in the house as the project drew to a close. My family, including my parents, Hilda and Pat, also experienced the illness and the surgery with me and in many ways would be as able to write a book as I am. For all their encouragement I am very grateful.

I am a professional academic and a number of colleagues have been particularly helpful over the years. David May of Dundee University was instrumental in getting me to formulate the personal experience of illness in scientific terms, Ray Fitzpatrick of Oxford University helped translate a research project into a book. In David and Ray respectively as mentor and editor I have been very fortunate. Several other colleagues have made encouraging noises along the way, notably Gareth Williams of Manchester University, Ruth Pinder of Brunel University, Hilary Thomas of Cambridge University, Priscilla Alderson in London, Neil McKeganey, John Anderson, Patrick West, Rex Taylor, Andrew Boddy, Robin Knill-Jones and Andrew Tannahill in home base in Glasgow, and Sarah Cunningham-Burley in Edinburgh.

The research on which this book is based was not funded through public sources. It is perhaps a sign of the times that I had to find private funds from industry to undertake the work. I am very grateful therefore to Hollister Ltd, Salt & Son, Simcare, Convatec, and Clinimed Ltd. In particular Ms Jean Marceau, Mr Peter Salt, Mr

John Cottrell and Mr Hugh Brady were prepared to support scientific work when it was far from clear that any definite outcome would follow.

Several other individuals have advised or helped and I would like to record my thanks to Barbara Wade then of the RCN, Professor Brian Brooke, Margaret McBride, Eleanor Russell, Caron Butler, Andy Malone, Cameron McDonald, Jim Attree, Charles Abraham, Jan Ireland, Norma Ballany, Archie Pagan, Maureen Munns, Carol Gordon, Kathy Staddle, Chris Penney, George Fenton, Jim McEwen, Jean Leiper and Jean Money.

Finally, there would be no research without subjects. My warmest appreciation goes to the unacknowledged and anonymous fifty men and women who had had ulcerative colitis or who had it and were about to undergo surgery to cure it. They shared with me in the most intimate and revealing ways, their struggles, their disasters, their shame and their embarrassments. They also shared their triumphs and their successes. I have tried to report their experiences as accurately as possible in this book. Their stories represent the real experience of coping with ulcerative colitis and colectomy as described here.

Editors' preface

Ulcerative colitis is a disease that assaults the individual in particularly distressing and disturbing ways. Initial symptoms are unpleasant, disruptive, embarrassing and difficult to explain. When eventually individuals seek medical care, the examinations and investigations that lead to diagnosis are also distressing. Eventually symptoms may become so overwhelming that patient and doctor have to consider surgical rather than drug therapy. The need to accept the idea of surgery imposes new demands on the individual, as the severity of symptoms are weighed against the threat of ileostomy and its consequences. Once surgery is over the individual has to adjust to the quite different body produced by ileostomy. A number of new and vital competencies have to be acquired, particularly learning how to wear, use and change a stoma appliance. The individual has to gain technical mastery over bodily functions others take for granted. In addition he or she also wants to continue normal life with a stoma, coping with potential embarrassments and disruptions in everyday interactions as well as potential threats to more intimate relationships.

Michael Kelly has written a volume which demonstrates beyond doubt the value of sociological and psychological concepts in drawing out the general truths to be gained from patients' accounts of such intimate and personal sources of suffering. To examine how individuals cope with a disease involving the most taboo of problems such as frequent and unpredictable diarrhoea pre-surgically or acceptance and management of a stoma post-surgically, he draws out the relevance of classic concepts of self, identity and coping from the social sciences. To do this, Michael Kelly pays close attention to the meanings of illness experience for individuals. For many individuals the experience of colitis is a source of anger and resentment, and surgery with all of its consequences a traumatic challenge. Nevertheless, post-surgical life was, for the vast majority of individuals interviewed by Kelly, viewed positively and with hope and contrasted very favourably with their pre-surgical state. The complex ways in which the individual comes through the enormously varied challenges to live a full and independent life with ileostomy is analytically and sharply delineated in this account. Michael Kelly has drawn on a broad and rich understanding of the social sciences as well as his own personal experience of colitis to achieve this invaluable contribution to our series concerned with the experience of illness.

Ray Fitzpatrick and
Stanton Newman, 1992

Chapter one

The background

The basic medical facts about ulcerative colitis may be described very simply: it is a non-specific inflammatory condition of the mucous membrane of the large bowel and rectum (Bouchier, 1977: 136), which tends to appear in early adulthood (Goligher *et al.*, 1980: 689). Its causes are unclear, but its pathology is well defined (Morson and Dawson, 1979: 331). The core symptoms are diarrhoea with passage of blood and mucus, abdominal pain, loss of energy and weight, and raised temperature (Goligher *et al.*, 1980: 701). There are a variety of complications which may include perforation of the bowel, and cancer.

For the people who have this illness there are social and psychological dimensions to the disease far beyond the pathology of the specific lesion. The ability to function socially can be severely undermined. Episodes of unpredictable diarrhoea punctuate all life's activities: from eating, through sleeping, to sex. Life may, at times, literally revolve around going to the toilet, or at least being near a toilet in case the need to evacuate arises. The unpredictability of the diarrhoea may render even an otherwise innocuous situation terrifying. A simple stroll in the country, a journey on a bus, a weekend away at friends can all be ruined, not only by the diarrhoea but also by the fear that it might overtake the person at any moment and cause mess and embarrassment.

However, there is more than just embarrassment associated with this disease. Young adults are not supposed to soil themselves: in infancy and in old age it might be accepted, but in the prime of life it is quite unacceptable. One of the most basic human functions is control of the bowel and control is undermined by this disease. The grown man and woman who suffers from this condition is in a situation which may at times resemble that of a child, and whose strategies for containing the diarrhoea may involve using nappies, pads or other aids, all of which may serve to reinforce loss of adult social status.

There is no medical cure for ulcerative colitis at present. There are, however, surgical cures, the most common of which involves the complete removal of the colon, anus and rectum and the diversion of the ileum through the skin to produce a new artificial anus called an ileostomy. This new opening has no muscular control, so the patient becomes permanently incontinent of faeces. After the operation the patient will have to wear, for the rest of his or her life, a plastic or rubber bag to collect digestive waste matter.

For many patients the operation may seem like jumping out of the frying pan into the fire. The operation leaves them free of disease so long as there have not been any malignant complications. However, the cure all but destroys the wholeness and the symmetry of the body. They have to wear an appliance (a bag) which may be bulky and appear to be visible under their clothing. They may have difficulties with the wearing of this appliance. Sometimes bags come off; not infrequently they leak. The person with the ileostomy may feel that his or her whole body has been violated and damaged.

However, most patients come through the experience reasonably well. Most get back to something like a normal existence, and most lead quite ordinary lives post-operatively. Nevertheless, the experience of the illness and surgery can be quite devastating and this book highlights these things as well as the problems of long-term adjustment.

Before proceeding to consider the main elements in the experience of illness and surgery, this chapter describes the basic medical details of colitis.

Epidemiology and aetiology

Ulcerative colitis was first described by Wilks in 1859 (Wilks and Moxon, 1875). In some ways the name ulcerative colitis is misleading because the term ulcerative does not mean the existence of discrete ulcers in all patients, and the rectum as well as the colon is involved in most cases (Goligher et al., 1980: 689). It is predominantly a disease of young adulthood but can appear at any age (Morson and Dawson, 1979: 525). The annual incidence of diagnosed ulcerative colitis is 5 to 10 per 100,000 of population in the United States and northern Europe. The prevalence is 100 per 100,000 of population (Goodman and Sparberg, 1978: 7–8). The disease is more common among whites than blacks and is between three and five times more common among Jews than Gentiles.

There is some evidence of a tendency for colitis to run in families (Binder *et al.*, 1966: 52–4; Allan and Hodgson, 1986: 302–3; Mahida, 1987: 161). However, it does not do so invariably in a direct way. The most common familial pattern is for the disease to affect two or more siblings or other first degree relatives (Kirsner, 1973: 559; Lewkonia and McConnell, 1976: 236). On the other hand the number of husbands and wives with the disease is minuscule. The evidence thus points to a genetic element in the causation. There is some supporting evidence for this on the basis of association with other diseases. Whether the genetic action is one of predisposition, susceptibility or response to something in the environment, remains a matter for future medical research (Kirsner, 1973: 557–71; Lewkonia and McConnell, 1976: 241; Mayberry, 1985: 970–1; Mahida, 1987: 168).

The idea of a relationship between personality type and colitis and the relationship between stress and the onset of the disease has received considerable attention over the years. It is now agreed that the early psychoanalytic work on colitis was unreliable. However, more recent work by psychologists using standard personality tests (like the Minnesota Multiphasic Personality Interview, the Eysenck Personality Inventory and the Cornell Medical Index) has proved rather better at finding relationships (Whitehead and Schuster, 1985: 132–7). Whitehead and Schuster, after reviewing the literature, concluded that people with ulcerative colitis show more obsessive-compulsive behaviours, may be shy and inhibited and may be overly dependent on their mothers or other care givers. However, these personality traits are not universal enough to be regarded as pathogenic and they are not usually severe enough to be considered abnormal (Whitehead and Schuster, 1985: 137). A controlled study of the association between ulcerative colitics and psychiatric illness showed that patients with colitis had a similar incidence of psychiatric problems to patients with non-gastro-intestinal chronic disorders. There was a marginally higher level of obsessive symptomatology but little evidence of major psychiatric problems (Helzer *et al.*, 1982). Goligher notes that the odd behaviour sometimes exhibited by people with colitis tends to subside after surgery and suggests that the disturbance is therefore a consequence rather than a cause of the disease (Goligher *et al.*, 1980: 691).

The currently favoured view of the origins of ulcerative colitis is that it is an immunological response to antigens (Allan and Hodgson, 1986: 303–6; Mahida, 1987: 164–7). However, which particular antigens are involved is a matter of debate. Among patients with ulcerative colitis some abnormal features in certain immunological tests appear (Goodman and Sparberg, 1978: 13). The mechanism involves some external agent (for example, a virus or a food additive) entering the bowel and having immunological cross reactivity within it. It has a chemical structure that is dissimilar enough from the body to elicit an immune response (antibody development) but similar enough for the antibodies that are developed also to attack the body tissue. Later, any factor that elicits an immune response (for example, bacterial infection or stress) produces an exaggerated response that attacks the bowel itself (Whitehead and Schuster, 1985: 131).

Sometimes organs and joints other than the gut are involved in ulcerative colitis and conditions such as arthritis, ankylosing spondylitis, erythema nodosum, pyoderma gangrenosum, iritis, episcleritis and hepatitis may also occur. There is some argument as to whether ulcerative colitis is a generalized disease affecting the whole body, or whether 'distant' complications are secondary to the main disease in the bowel. The weight of opinion seems to favour the idea that complications are distant and secondary because they are nearly always cured when the bowel is removed surgically (Goligher *et al.*, 1980: 692). The idea that antigen–antibody complexes mediate the inflammation in ulcerative colitis is attractive and could explain not only the colonic inflammation, but also its association with extra-intestinal manifestations (Mahida, 1987: 164).

Symptoms, course, outlook and complications

Although a few patients have constipation with small amounts of bleeding, usually the most obvious complaint is diarrhoea. The violence of the diarrhoea depends on the extent of the disease in the bowel (Goodman and Sparberg, 1978: 31–4). In some cases it is only mild, but in others there may be as many as twenty or more motions in 24 hours. This may lead to virtual incontinence, not from the failure of the sphincter muscles but from the exhaustion and weakness which prevent the sufferer from getting to the lavatory.

One of the most characteristic features of the diarrhoea is the sense of urgency of defecation which the patient experiences: only a few seconds warning in the case of an acute attack. The sense of urgency has the effect of overriding normal bowel control. Patients may experience colicky pain and usually the greater the lesions, the greater the pain. Continuous severe pain may indicate bowel perforation (Goligher *et al.*, 1980: 701). Severe pain is not inevitably a prominent feature of colitis, although cramps may be a daily occurrence relieved only by going to the toilet (Goodman and Sparberg, 1978: 34–6).

In all forms of ulcerative colitis, even the mild ones, there is an impairment of general health and well-being, and employment may become impossible. In acute cases the sufferer will be bedridden and grossly debilitated. Weight loss of 20–30 kg. is not uncommon in these circumstances. During remission the general health of the patient tends to improve, but sufferers are frequently thin and emaciated and with each recurrence their general health and appearance declines (Mallet *et al.*, 1978).

Three forms of colitis have been distinguished: chronic relapsing, chronic continuing and active fulminating colitis. Chronic relapsing colitis is the most common consisting of an initial attack, spontaneous remission, symptom freedom or mild symptoms and exacerbation of symptoms. The same cycle may be repeated many times. In chronic continuous colitis the symptoms are of moderate severity but are continuous. Active fulminating colitis is a very acute form of disease, producing rapid, extensive and sometimes fatal deterioration (Goligher *et al.*, 1980: 209–11).

The prognosis of ulcerative colitis is to some extent unpredictable. However, the age and the onset of the first attack is a significant prognostic feature, the elderly being most at risk from fatalities. If a patient survives an initial attack he or she has a very high chance of having another attack within three years. The severity and mortality of subsequent attacks are determined by the extent of the colitis and the patient's age. Ulcerative colitis is only very rarely a disease that remits completely and once someone has an attack, even if it goes into remission, he or she remains diseased and is at risk of further attacks (Goodman and Sparberg, 1978: 4; Jewell, 1987: 171–5).

There are important complications in ulcerative colitis. These are: perforation of the bowel, acute dilatation of the colon (toxic megacolon), haemorrhage, stricture of the colon, polyposis, fistula, and cancer of the colon and rectum (Goligher *et al.*, 1980: 712–20). Toxic megacolon, haemorrhage and cancer carry grave prognoses. The incidence of cancer rises progressively with the length of history of the colitis and lies between 3 and 5 per cent of all cases (Goligher *et al.*, 1980: 720; Morson and Dawson, 1979: 534). The greater the amount of bowel affected by the disease, the greater the likelihood of the development of cancer (Goligher *et al.*, 1980: 720). Patients with symptoms of chronic continuous disease seem more prone to cancer than those with the relapsing type (Morson and Dawson, 1979: 534). Cases where the colitis begins in childhood are at greatest risk (Goligher *et al.*, 1980: 721). In one prospective study of colitis it was demonstrated that there was no increased risk of cancer until the patient had had symptoms for ten years. Between ten and twenty years the excess risk was twenty-three times that expected in the general population (Lennard-Jones *et al.*, 1977).

Medical care for colitis is well defined. Close co-operation between physicians and pathologists is recommended in conjunction with an initially conservative attitude to treatment. Patients are followed up with annual sigmoidoscopy, and rectal biopsies. If the cell nuclei do not show any evidence of dysplasia it is assumed that the patient can safely be left for conservative management for another twelve months. If, however, the biopsies turn out to be positive and show undoubted dysplasia, the biopsies should be repeated three or four months later and if these are also positive, operation should be considered (Goligher *et al.*, 1980: 727). This is a quite complicated clinical judgement because the speed of progress from pre-cancerous to malignant appearance is variable.

Examination, diagnosis and medical treatment

The examining physician will use rectal examination to identify ulcerative colitis. There are various techniques for rectal investigation including proctoscopy and sigmoidoscopy. Proctoscopy and sigmoidoscopy involve the use of instruments to examine the mucosa. During sigmoidoscopy biopsies may be taken to analyse the microscopic processes of colitis. Fibre-optic colonoscopes allow for deep visual inspection of the bowel and are combined with biopsies. Barium enema is another technique. Barium is drained into the patient via the rectum and then X-ray photographs are taken.

Abdominal examination may reveal tenderness in a patient in whom the diagnosis is already established.

Goligher and his collaborators considered that the diagnosis of ulcerative colitis was very simple. 'The symptoms are highly suggestive and confirmation is readily obtained by sigmoidoscopy and barium enema examination' (1980: 707). Other authors, however, stress the difficulties in differentiating ulcerative colitis from Crohn's disease (Myers and Hightower, 1968: 920; Kirsner, 1973: 569; Morson and Dawson, 1979: 542–9).

There is no simple medical therapy for ulcerative colitis and the physician seeks out spontaneous remission. Moreover, the precise effects of medical therapy are difficult to evaluate because of the cyclical pattern of the disease. Two drugs are the mainstays of treatment: corticosteroids and sulphasalazine (salazopyrin).

Corticosteroids seem to be of most use in first attacks: their effectiveness apparently declines thereafter (Goligher et al., 1980: 230–1). The major problem with corticosteroids is side-effects, the development of which more or less parallels the anti-inflammatory effectiveness of the drug. The principal side effects are 'moon-faced' visage, facial hair, thinning of scalp hair, truncal obesity, wasting of limb muscles and acne. Steroids can also interfere with the physiology of sexual activity as well as of the body's healing mechanisms. Steroids may induce mood alterations. The effects of steroids may thus complicate the assessment of the disease itself. The administration of steroids has an inhibiting effect on the hypothalmo–pituitary–adrenal axis, and the longer the use, the greater the damage, particularly to the patient's ability to respond adequately to acute illness.

Sulphasalazine is more effective in mild and moderate ulcerative colitis than in severe forms. The sulphasalazine acts as an anti-inflammatory agent. It does not cure the colitis but helps to prevent flare-ups. Sulphasalazine does have a number of possible side-effects including nausea, vomiting, skin rashes, blood dyscrasias, joint and muscle pains and headaches (Goodman and Sparberg, 1978: 122–3; Hawkey and Hawthorne, 1988).

Surgical treatment

The operation currently favoured by many surgeons is panproctocolectomy and ileostomy. This operation involves the removal of the entire large bowel from the ileum close to the ileocaecal valve, down to and including the rectum. A combined abdominal and perineal approach is used (Goodman and Sparberg, 1978: 150). The operation is extensive and major. It requires a long left-sided incision from the pubis to the costal margin. The colon is removed by a process known as right and left hemi-colectomy. The rectum is taken out by synchronous combined abdomino-perineal excision. Then the ileostomy is constructed.

This is an extremely delicate and tricky part of the procedure. The site of the ileostomy should be such that there is an area of smooth flat skin all around to which the bag may be stuck. It is suggested that the ileostomy should be placed on the anterior abdominal wall in the right lower quadrant. It ought to be low enough for the patient to wear a belt to support the ileostomy appliance if necessary, but high enough for the bag to hang unobstructed in the right iliac fossa so that the flange of the ileostomy appliance does not impinge on the iliac crest and is clear of the umbilicus (Goodman and Sparberg, 1978: 151). The ileostomy itself should project some 2.5 to 4 cm. (Goligher et al., 1980: 757). The standard type of ileostomy is known as the Brooke ileostomy (after its originator). The stoma is constructed so that the whole thickness of the last centimetre or two of the ileum is everted, and its cut edge is stitched to the separate skin incision used for making the ileostomy.

In the last twenty years new surgical techniques have been devised. These include the continent or reservoir ileostomy. Here an internal pouch is constructed out of the ileum with a nipple valve to allow periodic emptying by the insertion of a catheter. Unfortunately, there is a high incidence of valve failure and the procedure has now been largely abandoned. Another procedure favoured by some surgeons is total colectomy with ileorectal anastomosis. This entails connecting the ileum to the upper rectum after the colon is removed. The risk of malignant disease of the rectum remains, so regular long-term follow-up is required. During the last ten years a number of surgeons have been carrying out restorative proctocolectomy with a pelvic ileal reservoir. The principle of this procedure is that the colon and rectum are removed to the level of the pelvic floor muscles (leaving the anal sphincter mechanism intact). The lining of the short length of rectum remaining is removed leaving only a rectal muscular cuff. An ileal reservoir or pouch is then constructed and the apex of this pouch is pulled down through the rectal muscular cuff and stitched to the anal canal. After this procedure frequency of defecation is approximately four to six times per day with patients having to wake up once per night. Over 90 per cent of patients in one study preferred this pouch, despite its problems, to a stoma because of an improvement in social and sexual image, self-confidence, cleanliness and freedom at work (see Kock, 1971; Jones et al., 1977; Parks and Nicholls, 1978; Pezim and Nicholls, 1985; Williamson and Mortensen, 1986; Keighley et al., 1987).

It is widely recognized in medical and nursing circles that making a recommendation for total colectomy is a very serious matter (Roy et al., 1970: 77; The Lancet, 1982: 1079; Rideout, 1987: 254–6). In principle the medical arguments are straightforward. In practice it is the psychological response of the patient which is difficult to assess and deal with. Goligher argues that the commonest reason for resorting to surgery is the intractability of the disease and the consequent chronic invalidism, resulting in such poor health that the only route back to health is via the operation (Goligher et al., 1980: 739). However, when the colitis is mild and confined to the rectum, and symptoms are at a low level, then surgery should not be considered (Watts et al., 1966: 1006; Goligher et al., 1968: 225). There is a wide range of manifestation of colitis between these two extremes and in the cases which are neither good nor bad the decision to recommend surgery is more difficult. Degree and severity of attacks, extent of the colitis and the age of the patient would all be taken into consideration by the surgeon (Goligher et al., 1980: 739–40).

In the case of a severe attack it is suggested that after three or four days where no unequivocal signs of remission are evident, immediate surgical intervention is important (Goligher et al., 1968: 228; 1980: 742). A fever of 38.3°C, more than twelve stools daily, abdominal pain and profuse bleeding are recommended by Bouchier (1977: 146) as the key markers for surgical intervention. Emergency intervention may also be required if there is a danger of toxic megacolon, haemorrhage or perforation of the bowel (Goodman and Sparberg, 1978: 148–9). Over the years, as operative mortality has improved and post-operative complications lessened election for surgery has become much more common than emergency procedures (Daly and Brooke, 1967: 62).

Goodman and Sparberg argue that there are five relative indications for colectomy which summate with each other for recommendation for surgery. These are persistence of symptoms, continuing blood loss, peripheral manifestations of ulcerative colitis, pointers to a particular predisposition to develop cancer (long history, young age of onset, chronic disease activity) and the presence of epithelial dysplasia in biopsy (Goodman and Sparberg, 1978: 150). Since ulcerative colitis may cause physical retardation in children, it is important, they argue, to consider the operation for such cases to help to ensure healthy growth. Finally, severe local abscesses, fissures and fistulas are also indications for surgery (Goligher et al., 1980: 740–2).

Post-operative concerns

In the immediate post-operative period there are a number of possible complications which may occur after total colectomy. These include skin irritation (caused by the fluids discharging from the stoma); ileostomy dysfunction (caused by partial obstruction of the ileostomy opening); haemorrhage; wound infection; and intra-abdominal infection (Ritchie, 1971: 532–3). There may be cardio-pulmonary complications especially in smokers. Patients with ulcerative colitis are particularly prone to potentially fatal deep venous thrombosis and pulmonary embolism (Goodman and Sparberg, 1978: 156). Post-operative complications are much more common in patients undergoing emergency surgery than those undergoing elective surgery (Goligher et al., 1968: 294; Ritchie, 1971: 531). On the whole it is estimated that about two-thirds of patients have no significant post-operative complications (Valkamo, 1981: 261). Hospital mortality for this operation is about 3 per cent overall, urgent and emergency operations carrying a higher risk than the elective procedure (Ritchie, 1971: 531; Valkamo, 1981: 8).

In the longer term the post-operative problems revolve not around the disease or the surgery but around learning to live with the appliance. There are many different types of appliance, coming in various shapes and sizes, and involving a range of fixing methods. They are made of plastic and (less frequently these days) rubber materials. Ileostomy bags have to be drained perhaps four or five times a day. A bag has to be replaced by a new one every four or five days or sometimes longer. Some appliances are transparent, others are opaque. Usually someone with an ileostomy will wear a cotton cover over the appliance. Cotton tends to be more comfortable than either plastic or rubber when worn against the skin. Cotton covered appliances also fit more snugly under clothing.

Probably the most frequent long-term metabolic complication is the tendency towards chronic, though usually symptomless, sodium and water depletion (*The Lancet*, 1982: 1079; Cummings, 1988). There are a number of other more significant longer-term complications. Stenosis, which is the narrowing of the channel in the ileostomy, is much less common nowadays than it once was, as a result of the introduction of the Brooke ileostomy. Obstructions caused by adhesions can be a problem. Skin irritation is another extremely common difficulty, arising as a consequence of the intestinal contents, and in particular the pancreatic juices, coming into contact with the peristomal skin. This causes rawness. Contact dermatitis may occur at the interface of skin and appliance. Once skin problems have become established they can be particularly difficult to cure because of the presence of the appliance preventing healing and the fact that without an appliance the person with an ileostomy will be rendered immobile because of incontinence. A majority of people with ileostomies seem to suffer some skin problems (Fussell, 1976: 659; Mayberry and Rhodes, 1978: 959; Valkalmo, 1981: 33; Finan, 1988: 1250–1).

The absence of a colon may leave the ileostomy patient vulnerable to infectious gastroenteritis. The accompanying diarrhoea and vomiting can be severely debilitating because of dehydration (Goodman and Sparberg, 1978: 166). Profuse discharge and dehydration can be caused by blockages of food. This may occur where food has been only partially chewed or digested, or foods high in fibre have been over-consumed to the point of forming a bolus.

Prolapse, meaning the ileum sliding through the abdominal wall, and retraction of the stoma can be troublesome for some patients and along with the development of hernias, abscesses and fistulae may be indications for further surgery to reposition the stoma (Goodman and Sparberg, 1978: 155–65). Another long-term complication is slow healing of the perineal wound with perhaps as many as one quarter of patients having this problem (Myers and Hightower, 1968: 922). Weight gain is a problem for some patients (Kirkpatrick *et al.*, 1979: 203). It has been claimed that ileostomists are particularly prone to develop kidney stones but the evidence seems to be equivocal (Goligher *et al.*, 1980: 792; Morowitz and Kirsner, 1981: 374; *The Lancet*, 1982: 1079).

11

For patients about to undergo surgery there is, in most western countries, a considerable infrastructure of support available in addition to doctors. There are specialists in stoma therapy called enterostomal therapists or stoma care nurses. These have particular training and qualifications to undertake the work. The companies that manufacture the appliances frequently provide support and assistance in the form of patient education leaflets and books and sometimes provide stoma care services themselves.

Patients also help themselves. There are flourishing self-help groups and associations with local, national, and even international organizations. These work in different ways in different countries, but their stated aims are usually the sharing of experiences, the provision of information, and sometimes also pressure group activity, lobbying and social support (Brooke, 1986). The self-help groups sometimes work closely with the medical and nursing professions, and some support scientific and other research endeavours.

Conclusion

This chapter has, with the help of a number of standard texts, sketched out the basic medical and surgical details of ulcerative colitis. Readers wanting to pursue these things in more detail are referred particularly to Goligher *et al.*, (1980), Morson and Dawson (1979) and Brooke (1986). But the experience of colitis, as with any disorder, is not simply a matter of medical fact. The illness has an effect on sufferers, on their families, their work, and their relationships with others. What the remainder of the book deals with are these issues.

The bloody diarrhoea marks a break with normal body functioning. It is a symptom that cannot be easily ignored either by sufferers or by their families and friends, as they begin to make sudden exits from social situations or perhaps avoid them altogether. If the person self-soils, even if others do not know, the challenge to the idea that he or she is a competent adult can be considerable. However, the implications go beyond mere social disgrace. The disease is statistically most likely to appear when someone is entering adulthood or is in the prime of life. He or she is likely to be starting or to have recently begun, to take on adult roles (work, marriage, parenthood). The onset of the disease may therefore have dire effects in the short and long term on the adult's ability to support dependants or develop a career.

Additionally the illness may have particularly threatening connotations if, and when, surgery is recommended. Not only is it a major procedure in itself, involving extensive tissue damage, but also it is an operation which in a very important sense transforms the body. One of the most basic and obvious of human biological functions, the evacuation of waste matter, is radically altered and its site moved. The real and imagined responses of others to this have to be considered. The illness and its surgery are about faeces and their management. Faeces, diarrhoea and stomas are the stuff of symbolism, swearing, joking, taboo and dirt. The cultural overlay of these things will also be important.

People who have colitis and those who acquire an ileostomy have partially, or totally, lost control of their bodies. Coming to terms with that loss and finding ways of coping with the illness and with the surgery are the essence of the experience of both colitis and colectomy.

The data: a note

Where original data are presented in the following chapters they are drawn from fifty interviews which were conducted with people who either already had had a colectomy as a consequence of ulcerative colitis, or who were ill and were soon to undergo surgery. In all cases subjects either had or were to have panproctocolectomy and ileostomy. None of the subjects had the other types of surgical techniques. Sometimes multiple interviews were conducted pre- and post-operatively. The interviews did not rely on a structured schedule because the purpose was not to gather quantitative or pre-coded information for statistical analysis. Rather a series of prompts were used to guide the discussion in order to allow the subjects to talk freely and wide-rangingly about their experiences. The objective was not to test a particular scientific hypothesis nor to collect large numbers of cases. The aim was to encourage the ordinary men and women who had had colitis to talk about their triumphs and tragedies, their disasters and their successes. I wanted as authentic a picture as possible of what it was like to have colitis.

Thus I opted to use what is usually known as a qualitative methodology. All the interviews were tape-recorded. All subjects knew that I myself had had colitis and that I had an ileostomy. I would start the interviews by asking the subjects to describe how their trouble first began. Many of the people would begin by saying that they had nothing very interesting to say, but after a little encouragement, would speak at great length. I seldom used less than sixty minutes' worth of tape and often considerably more.

The evenings spent with the subjects were most enjoyable. After arriving at each subject's house, where most of the interviews were conducted, I would usually be shown to the 'best' room. There I would explain the purposes of my study and say a little about myself. Then I would switch the tape recorder on and let the subjects tell their stories. When they had finished I would use a check list to see if there were any points they had not covered and ask them if they wanted to make any further comments. Sometimes spouses or children would join us for all or part of the evening. Almost invariably the subjects were extremely hospitable and I ate my way through cakes, chocolate biscuits and consumed gallons of tea and coffee.

The interviews were transcribed by me. The method of analysis of the voluminous pages of transcription was as follows. I originally constructed a list of broad topic areas of interest which seemed germane to the experience of colitis. Not unnaturally my own experience played an important part in determining this first list. My feeling was that rather than trying to submerge my own experience it was better to acknowledge it quite deliberately at this stage. However, I was also familiar with some of the scientific literature on the experience of colitis – notably Reif's work (Reif, 1973a, 1973b) – as well as the accounts which appeared in the journal of the Ileostomy Association. These attuned me to issues beyond my own personal experience. I had read widely some of the major sociological accounts of life with chronic illness such as Wiener (1975), Bury (1982), Locker (1983) and Williams (1984). I also knew Beatrice Wright's (1983) major psychological study of the experience of disability. These sources together allowed me to draw up a reasonably comprehensive list of issues or themes.

However, as I listened to the tapes, new themes emerged and new ideas suggested themselves and these joined the topic list. The transcriptions were cross-referenced to as many categories or issues as they seemed to fit. This was done manually using a card index system. Eventually after recording and rethinking, a range of ideas emerged, which form the basis both of the original research report (Kelly, 1990) and this book. The central theme was coping with illness and surgery.

The fifty people who were interviewed are not in any sense a statistically representative group. Therefore, no attempt is made to argue that the experiences described here are statistically significantly different from the behaviour manifested by non-colitics or patients undergoing other major surgery. It is, however, my contention that these fifty cases are themselves sufficiently similar, and that the themes and issues which vex these people have sufficient in common, to make the case that a non-sufferer, a carer, a medical practitioner, a nurse, or a relative will learn something about the experience of colitis from these accounts. I would also contend that what follows would ring true to anyone who has colitis or who has been cured of it by the operation.

The fifty people were in fact an opportunity sample. They were drawn from a number of sources. The two practising stoma therapists working in the area where I was based both co-operated. Between them they had the most complete list of local ostomy patients. They willingly agreed to help and suggested names of patients whom I might see. The Ileostomy Association was also a great help. I met with the two nearest local secretaries and got their permission to approach their members. Circumstances dictated that in one case I used a snowball technique, that is, getting the person I was interviewing to suggest any other people I might interview, and then contacting them. In the other case I went along to one of the regular meetings and appealed for volunteers and collected names and addresses at the end of the meeting. Naturally, therefore, my sample is biased towards volunteers who are members of the voluntary associations, and who are prepared to talk to a relative stranger about their problems. Non-joiners, social isolates, and others are correspondingly underrepresented. I was also introduced to several subjects via the local surgeons who, aware of my sampling problems, were keen for me to see a good cross-section of people. Their recommendations helped balance some of the more gregarious volunteers. In the absence of good local epidemiological data about the disease or the surgical cases and the practical impossibility of gathering a continuous series of patients coming through all the local hospitals dealing with the disease (I was fully employed as a teacher all the time I gathered the data and was not

15

free during the day to go to out-patient clinics for example), my opportunity sample seemed the best available option. Undoubtedly some 'purists' will find the methodology weak and woolly. I hope, however, for all its apparent scientific weakness, it gives a revealing insight into the world of colitis and colectomy.

It should be noted that five of the fifty subjects were excluded from the final analysis, one because of tape malfunction, two because of clear medical histories and surgery contra-indicative of colitis, one was lost to follow-up and one was a youngster whose responses were made for him by his mother, who sat in on the interview.

Of the 45 analysed responses there were 30 women and 15 men. The average age was 42.5 years (women 39 and men 48). There were 25 married respondents (16 women and 9 men), 15 single people (10 women and 5 men), 2 female divorcees, 2 widows and 1 widower. Of the 30 who were or had been married, 23 had children and some had grandchildren and great-grandchildren. Thirty-one subjects were in paid employment or full-time education, 6 were retired, 4 described themselves as housewives, and 4 said they were unemployed. The respondents were drawn from all occupational groups in the Registrar General's Classification of Occupations.

Where extracts from the interviews are used, they have been slightly edited, and punctuated, for ease of reading. The respondents' names have been changed, and some features in their stories have been altered, to preserve anonymity. In some cases composite subjects have had to be 'invented' in order to make sure that personal identity markers were completely obscured. This has been done as far as possible in the spirit of the original transcripts.

Chapter two

The start of the trouble

Something out of the ordinary

The starting-point for the analysis of the experience of colitis is with the onset of the disease. More specifically, the focus is on the first recognition by the sufferer that something unusual, or out of the ordinary, is happening. The characteristic response to the initial symptoms of colitis seems to be one of uncertainty. For some people the onset is slow and insidious and there is a long transition from being healthy to being ill. The symptoms seem to creep up on the person, who may wonder if the problem is imaginary. The time of the start of the illness is uncertain. There are other people for whom there is a definite episode which heralds the start of the illness. But there is also some uncertainty because generally the episode is dismissed, initially at least, as a 'spot of tummy trouble', or as nothing more than diarrhoea brought upon by some dietary indiscretion or infection. Only in retrospect is the event seen as the start of a chronic illness.

Initial uncertainty gives way to clarity. Clarity comes from explanation. Among the subjects interviewed in this study, there was a strong tendency to explain the initial episode in benign terms. They saw their initial symptoms as harmless. This is perfectly reasonable. People like to think of themselves as normal, and slight deviations from normal body functioning are in themselves quite common. Having an 'upset tummy' or a 'touch of diarrhoea' would not usually be viewed by most people, as anything other than a transient nuisance. It is when such symptoms persist over a period of time that a reappraisal is necessary.

Andrew, a clerk in his late twenties, noticed a change in his bowel habit. The number of motions increased and he had passage of blood. He explained, 'It only lasted about five weeks. I had never heard of anybody having this sort of thing, and I thought it was piles or something. I also wondered if I was under stress at work. I thought maybe it would go away on its own.' Andrew found two not unreasonable explanations for what was happening, namely piles (a benign lay diagnosis) and stress. It was only with the next more severe episode, about six months later when it did not clear up of its own accord, that Andrew went to see a doctor.

Like Andrew, Harry (another office worker in his twenties) was able to pin-point when he noticed his first symptoms. He, however, was only able to ignore things for a couple of weeks. He was out playing golf: 'I had just finished the swing and I thought I'd passed wind, and I didn't give it a second thought until I was coming home. When I got home I noticed mucus on my underpants. I ignored it for about a week or a fortnight. But shortly after that I noticed blood. But that again didn't cause me much concern because I thought I was constipated. Only when this didn't clear up, did I go to the doctor's.'

Stella and Barbara were much less precise about when their trouble started. Stella, who was a housewife, said, 'I think it started when I was at school losing a lot of blood, at that time I was just ignorant, so I didn't think it was serious at all. I didn't tell anyone. It was only after I left school and went to work in a hospital that I realized there was anything wrong.' Barbara, who worked in a shop, said, 'I don't know when the symptoms actually first began. When I was at school I used to get diarrhoea a lot, so that it maybe stemmed from that, like worrying about exams and things like that.' Stella simply ignored her problems, while Barbara explained them away with reference to her anxiety about taking examinations. They both continued for several years untreated and it was only subsequent declines in health that stopped them both from earning a living, that led them to seek medical help.

Many other respondents had similar stories to tell about their initial contact with the problem. In behavioural terms changes were noted either immediately (Andrew and Harry) or gradually (Stella and Barbara). Whether immediate or gradual, the changes were ignored and discounted. All four subjects continued to think of themselves as basically healthy people rather than as being ill. They generated hypotheses about what might account for the persistence of the problem, such as piles, constipation and stress, all of which allow the episodes, even the chronic episodes, to be viewed as benign or irrelevant. Eventually all four were driven to make a medical consultation. The sociological question is what is it that changes the appraisal of these episodes from something benign which can be ignored, to something about which action must be taken.

'I must do something about this'

Eventually the person who is suffering with the symptoms of what turn out to be colitis decides that something must be done. Ignoring the problem, or hoping it will go away, or denying the existence of the symptoms, cease to be realistic ways of coping with the changes taking place in the body. In behavioural terms the changes have to be acknowledged for what they are, namely deviations from normal bowel function. A conscious decision has to be made that the deviation is not benign but something potentially harmful. This acknowledgement does not seem to be a sudden process. It does not appear to be the case that at one moment people with diarrhoea are pretending that they do not have it, or are explaining it away with reference to the meal they had the night before, and the next moment they decide they need to see a doctor. The transition is gradual and probably begins as soon as the signs are first noted. However, particular episodes can be powerful and traumatic catalysts in the process. The appearance of blood in the motion is a significantly alarming sign, which is sufficiently out of the ordinary to spur many people towards their doctor. Another key event can be the sudden loss of continence in embarrassing public circumstances. It is as if the individuals have been thinking about seeking help, but what they need is an unequivocal sign that they can legitimately do so. Seeking help may also have benefit for someone who has had an embarrassing episode of self-soiling. They 'medicalize' the problem by consulting a doctor and this provides an explanation of the event which may exonerate them from public disgrace. There are also cases where the trigger is simply the worsening of the symptoms themselves. The person passes a point where, in his or her own eyes, the benefits of trying to carry on as if nothing is wrong are outweighted by the costs – physical and emotional – of keeping going.

Some of the ways people tell the stories of the early part of their illnesses illustrate these ideas. First of all Simon, who worked away from home on oil rigs, had begun to notice that something wasn't quite right. 'I thought it was something I'd eaten, so I brushed it off. I knew I had some time off work to come, so I went home and I was hoping maybe a week or so away and it would clear up. But it didn't, so I went to the doctor. And he gave me these tablets which are standard for someone with a stomach upset. They didn't make any difference. Anyway I was still taking them when I went on holiday. And we were away five nights. But the diarrhoea got really bad. So we came straight back. And I went to the doctor and I said, "There's something wrong." I had this feeling it was going to be a hospital case.'

Simon tried to ignore his problem. He thought a few day's rest would help. In the end he felt overwhelmed by his symptoms. Interestingly, his doctor had initially helped put his mind at rest and made him feel better by treating it as a standard stomach upset. Then Simon had to return to the surgery and try and convince the doctor it was more than this and was a potential 'hospital case'.

Irene, a schoolteacher in her late twenties, took a different tack. She put her problems down to menstrual difficulties and generally overdoing things. 'I felt more tired than usual', she said; ' I felt as if I had period pains all the time. I'd never been bothered by period pains. I let it go for a little while. I thought it'll go away, it's just one of those things, possibly been overdoing things or doing too much hockey, or too much exercise, and it didn't go away so I went to my doctor.'

What had happened in both of these cases was that as the days and weeks passed, Simon and Irene were gradually forced to think of themselves differently. Social-psychologists and others sometimes use the term self-image to refer to the idea involved here. The social-psychological concept of self simply refers to the idea that each and every one of us carries around in our heads, ideas about who and what we are (Ball, 1972). For these subjects their self-image had to change from being a normal healthy person with a body that could be relied upon, to being someone who was sick.

This in turn creates another problem, because while the individuals may be beginning to think of themselves as people who have something wrong, they will seldom be confined to their sickbeds. They will be up and about, trying their best to carry on their life. In behavioural terms the private inner view (the self) of the person is of someone sick, but this is at odds with the way others see them. They still look normal, they still largely carry on as normal. From the point of view of people who are ill this produces tension because they feel obliged to try to carry on. Indeed they themselves may begin to doubt that they are ill. Their sense of self vacillates between health and illness.

Going along to a doctor and obtaining treatment is the public proclamation to others that the person is sick. Perhaps he or she gets a sickness absence certificate from the doctor, perhaps some treatment, or perhaps both; a person does, however, then have the legitimate right to relinquish some normal day-to-day responsibilities. This is not a process which he or she experiences in isolation. Close relatives and friends may be only too well aware of the difficulties that the diarrhoea is causing and may become embroiled in helping resolve the tension between being sick and carrying on as if nothing was wrong.

The sufferer has an impaired bodily function. That impairment is eventually recognized as something which prevents the fulfilment of some desired social, psychological or biological function. Attempts to explain this away as irrelevant or benign fail, and the sufferer, perhaps in conjunction with close family or friends, begins to see his or her symptoms as a threat. The task is to decide what to do about the threat. In modern western industrial societies the common-sense thing to do when threatened by something which is apparently sickness, or is defined as an illness, is to seek help. The most obvious source of help is the medical profession and, unsurprisingly, that is precisely where most of the subjects headed.

The important concept is threat. Two particularly important types of event are especially threatening for the person in the early stages of colitis: blood and incontinence. For some people it is the blood itself. Julie, a housewife, said, 'I went to the doctor. I said I was bleeding from the back passage and he said I had haemorrhoids. I got a course of iron tablets. When I said I was losing blood from the back passage I think the doctor thought it was a spot. Eventually I confided in my mother. In the end I used a little plastic potty, I thought when I need to I'll use that. Now all that I passed was blood. My mother got an awful shock. She was on to the doctor right away.' Julie, like Simon (above), had some difficulty convincing the doctor that there was a problem. Melanie, a trainee insurance broker, was someone else for whom blood constituted a vital sign. She said, 'Basically I am a very healthy person, I'd never really had anything wrong with me. And I started to notice some blood present when I went to the loo and that concerned me greatly. So I went to the doctor.'

However, for other people the threat derives not from the blood itself but what the blood might signify, the main worry being cancer. 'I just thought it was a bug, and after about two weeks I was getting worried. I was passing blood. And I thought, "It's cancer."' 'I thought I had cancer, I was prepared to believe at first that it was just nerves, and then it didn't improve and then there was blood.' These responses, from Gwen (a business woman) and Bernadette (a personal secretary), show a process from initial benign hypotheses – a bug in Gwen's case and nerves in Bernadette's – to the much more threatening possibility of cancer.

One last extract illustrates how sometimes it was being simply overwhelmed by the symptoms that was important. Mary, a trainee accountant, had already visited her GP and had been prescribed codeine phosphate. However, one morning her symptoms came to a head. 'Everyone had gone out. And I spent the whole of that morning sitting on the loo. I had never had diarrhoea like it before.' This she saw as a turning point in her illness.

'You really are ill'

So far in this chapter the concern has been with the way the person whose body has started to behave in unpredictable ways thinks and feels. The focus has been the shift in the way people think about themselves (their self) as they appraise threat in these bodily changes. However, human beings do not exist in vacuums. They have contact with other people. Moreover, other people have views and thoughts about them. The technical social-psychological term for this idea is identity. Identity is the public and knowable aspect of the individual. As the first part of the chapter has argued, in the early stages of this illness there may be a tension between the way sufferers see themselves (as people who are or who might be ill) and the way others see them (as people who are normal and well). There is a tension between self and identity. What has then to happen is for other people, or certain important other people like family, close friends and perhaps most important of all their doctors, to recognize them as being ill and ascribe them an identity as an ill person.

It will be remembered from Chapter one that this illness is

chronic, although its course is to some extent unpredictable. Sufferers may feel unwell but if they are unable to convince others that they are unwell, then attempts to come to terms with the illness may be more difficult. This is not a straightforward process. It is often slow and subject to delicate negotiation between patient and doctor.

That this is so is not surprising. Many people who consult their doctor because they have noticed something odd about their body's functioning either consult inappropriately, that is, they have misdiagnosed themselves, or present with self-limiting pathology. General practice is sometimes characterized as dealing with a large number of trivial problems like this. However, the symptoms of colitis are not self-limiting because a return to pre-morbid physiology is not likely, and because of the potential medical seriousness of the problem it is certainly not inappropriate to seek help. Nevertheless, in the early phases 'upset tummy', diarrhoea, even bleeding, can be accounted for medically as non-serious events. Sufferers are not infrequently told, 'There is a lot of it about' (as indeed there is); or piles, or nerves or some other benign condition is initially diagnosed.

This may leave patients with a difficulty because either their condition is untreated or it is treated inappropriately. The patients' own judgements are questioned. They have concluded that their symptoms are threatening enough to warrant seeking help, but then they are informed that they have acted inappropriately and that there is nothing to worry about. While this might provide reassurance, it can create still more uncertainty and alarm, especially if the symptoms persist. Martha, a school teacher, is a case in point. 'I began to feel unwell. Went to the GP who didn't examine me at all, and told me I was suffering from piles. The piles wouldn't go away and by this time it was really terribly painful. And I started to get really worried because I was losing blood. So I made an appointment with another doctor in the practice. She took me into the examination room, examined me straight away and within a week I was up the hospital.' Whereas Martha's initial diagnosis was the not uncommon one of piles, Gwen was thought to have typhoid. 'The doctor asked me if I had been abroad. He thought it was typhoid. Then they tested for everything.'

For both Martha and Gwen the identity as a legitimate patient was developed over a period of time. Both worried about the threat of cancer throughout the period that they experienced strange and discomforting symptoms. In the absence of information both came up with inaccurate but none the less extremely worrying lay explanations of what was happening. The threat increased throughout this period as, correspondingly, did their anxiety. Their anxiety was only relieved once the true diagnosis was made. For Martha and Gwen the change occurred fairly quickly, in a matter of months. For other patients the process sometimes took longer, the stress was correspondingly more drawn out and the relief of eventual diagnosis considerable.

Ulcerative colitis is a disease with definable pathology. It is also a social identity in which certain types of behaviours (mostly associated with the symptoms, like rushing to the toilet) are allowed or tolerated. In the same way as one might expect someone with arthritis to have difficulty in getting about, or someone with diabetes to be careful about what to eat, the person with colitis suddenly rushing out of the room becomes part of the routine of being ill. It can, however, only really become routine once the identity as a sick person is bestowed by other people. The diagnosis provides explanations both medically and socially to sufferers, and to their relatives and friends (assuming they decide to share it with them). The relief of finding out what the trouble really is is hardly surprising.

Unlike the cases of Martha and Gwen above, where the diagnosis provided relief, a diagnosis may sometimes provide a threat. The reason for this is loss of specialness. Some respondents admitted to enjoying having a mystery illness. Veronica, a computer operative, explained, 'It started when I was about ten and a half. It was blood rather than diarrhoea, and that went on until I was about thirteen. The doctor sent me to a gynaecologist, and they said they couldn't find anything wrong. From the age of fourteen, I found it quite difficult. The bouts were getting worse and closer together, and then I started having stomach pains. So I went to the doctor, who thought it was piles, but he sent me to a surgeon anyway, and they diagnosed what it was. And from then I went downhill.' While she had a mystery illness, Veronica seems to have enjoyed certain advantages and attentions which she evidently found quite satisfying. For her the diagnosis constituted the threat to that specialness.

Diagnosis

Many colitics find the means of arriving at diagnosis particularly unpleasant physically, socially and psychologically. Procedures such as barium enema and sigmoidoscopy are frequently experienced as humiliating and degrading. Julie explained, 'I got the appointment for the X-ray department, went in without a care in the world. I came out absolutely devastated. It was terrifying. I just didn't know what to expect. Previously I had had chest X-rays, but I hadn't a clue what was going to happen. You go into this place which has the revolving table and they pump all this stuff into you. It was ghastly.' Pauline, a nursery nurse, described a not uncommon experience. 'The last barium enema I had, they were busy taking pictures. The nurse hadn't blown up the balloon [the valve to keep the barium *in situ*] properly because it was hurting that much. I started to feel it coming out. The radiologist said it wouldn't. And out it came, it went everywhere. Oh what an embarrassment.' Lizzie, a factory worker, had a similar experience. 'I couldn't hold it in. As long as I was lying on my back I was able to clench it in. But once I turned on my side I just lost control. The whole lot came splashing out everywhere.'

Procedures such as sigmoidoscopy, and to a lesser extent colonoscopy, are frequently described no more favourably than barium enema. Patients find these procedures invasive, embarrassing and painful. Additionally the enema may be a particularly frightening experience because it takes place in a darkened room. The presence in the bowel of the barium creates a feeling of urgency of defecation, while the valve retaining the barium makes this impossible. The pain can be acute. Patients who have been through this experience often mention the fact that X-ray staff appear to be very unsympathetic.

In social terms the diagnostic procedures are also important. They reinforce the identity of the person as sick in a number of ways. They confirm the diagnosis which the physician suspects. They are critical events, because, from the patient's point of view, they provide certainty of diagnosis where perhaps before there was only vagueness. While this may be an inaccurate description when viewed from the medical perspective, especially if there are complicated issues of differential diagnosis involved, from the patient's point of view the first barium enema in particular marks a highly significant turning-point. It marks the time before which a return to normal health might be hoped for, but after which the person will be increasingly drawn into the medical orbit. This may be a welcome relief for some, a threat for others, but it is a point of personal significance none the less.

Resistance and acceptance

In spite of the fact that the medical profession has swung into action, in spite of the fact that it is usually the sufferers themselves who have initiated the contact with the medical services, in spite of the fact that often after a long and traumatic spell of illness and dealings with the medical profession a diagnosis has finally been reached, some people seem keen then to reject what has happened. They may try to resist their new identity as sick person in different ways. They may try to withdraw from medical treatment, they may try to seek out alternatives such as self-help or alternative healers. Sometimes this may be done in conjunction with conventional treatment, at other times it may be instead of it. Irene tried homoeopathy, or at least consulted someone calling himself a homoeopath. 'And the homoeopathic doctor asks dozens of questions about your whole person and things that have happened about the time of the illness, the onset of the illness. He tries to fit the illness into my persona and find out my dislikes and likes. He said he would have to analyse all the answers. So he tried this remedy and I believed in it. I saw him regularly and he kept copious notes, and we changed the remedy quite often. And up to a point it was successful, but then at the worst stage he had to admit it wasn't doing me any good.' Rhona, a schoolgirl, self-helped. 'I used to try all those things to make you relax, herbal teas. I've still got a whole load of these things in the cupboard, all those cock-a-mee-mee things. None of them helped. I should just have left well enough alone.'

Patients may experiment with a range of alternative and complementary medicine in an attempt to find cures. The first line of treatment from conventional medicine is the attempt to stabilize the condition, so that the patient can get on with life *with* the disease. However, such regimens are not always very successful, when viewed from the patient's point of view. Seldom will the patient return to what he or she was like before the trouble began. What is on offer from the doctors may appear to be bland and unhelpful. The fact that this is the standard treatment is not especially reassuring. Worse, the drugs which the palliative treatment involves may produce unpleasant side-effects. Under the circumstances it seems perfectly logical to look elsewhere for help.

For most people who have colitis there comes a point when they have to accept the limits imposed upon them by their disease. This does not mean a point at which they give in to the disease. Nor is it the point when their illness is diagnosed. It is rather the point at which realization occurs that the disease is not going to go away of its own accord and is not going to be cured by the medical practitioner prescribing drugs. Many patients seem to function in the initial phases of their disease with an acute model of illness in their minds. Even if they have resisted the idea that they had anything wrong at first, eventually those who come into treatment make a decision that they need help. They approach the medical profession largely in the expectation that they will receive help. Of course they do, but the kind of help they get does not rid them of their problem. Instead it gives them an identity as a sick person. Moreover, this sickness is chronic. Gradually the patient has to come to terms with the chronicity of their disease. Indeed until they do, their strategies for living with their illness may be inappropriate (like trying to carry on without help) or may be more appropriate to a bout of acute sickness from which recovery might realistically be expected. Once the chronic nature of the problem is acknowledged coping can focus on the long-term effects of the illness.

It seems to be the case that particular events or turning-points or levels of disruption engendered by the symptoms are highly significant. The next couple of extracts provide examples of the level of disruption becoming a public matter. Kirsty, a legal student, said, 'I had days when I had diarrhoea and days when I was better. And I gradually got worse. As my exams approached I was more and more taken to bed and feeling rotten, and my friends were noticing I was rushing to the bathroom all the time. The week before my exams I was admitted to hospital.' After that there was no turning back.

Georgina, a young factory worker, expressed a similar idea: 'Some of my friends used to laugh. But I always got the feeling that nobody really understood how bad I was. They used to ring up, and I'd say I didn't want to go out. And if I did go out, I'd have to go home. So I would rush home and sit on the loo. I wouldn't drink and they'd be all sitting quite jolly and I'd be sitting there with a straight face just dying to get home.'

Both Kirsty and Georgina attempted to do normal, if rather different things: sit exams and go to the pub. Eventually they were swamped by their symptoms and had to admit to their difficulties. It was, however, a gradual process. For Martha, there was a much more sudden realization. When she talked about this episode she was still intensely embarrassed and distressed about it. 'I don't know how I coped, looking back, but I did, I managed to work and I wouldn't give in to it, I took the attitude that it's not going to beat me, I'm going to beat it, but in the end it did. The first really humiliating experience for me was when I realized things couldn't go on. I came out of work to meet my husband. I was waiting for him looking, in a shop window with the kids. I said to the kids, "Wait here for Dad, I have to go to the public toilets." I got there but I didn't make it, and I was so humiliated. There was absolutely no control. I couldn't tell anybody that this had happened to me. There was me in these public toilets having to take everything off. It was horrific. This was the big thing for me. Up until then I had always managed to get to the loo. There was nothing I could do, there was no control. I was desperate from then on. And I knew then that I couldn't go on with my life, like that.'

An even more extreme case was Donna, who said, 'I haemorr-haged badly in the night. I wakened up, and I was being sick out of one end, and there was blood gushing out of the other. I couldn't get out of bed, I was away. They whipped me into hospital.'

Conclusion

When the respondents' bodies began to behave in ways which were unusual, after the initial uncertainty the typical reaction was to explain what was happening in terms of common sense. Diarrhoea and tiredness are usual enough experiences, so it is hardly surprising that these patients behaved in the way they did. The common-sense explanations of over-indulgence, period pains, bugs, nerves, and stress all helped to maintain a sense that all was well because these things are part of normal human experience, and they pass. However, the symptoms of ulcerative colitis do not just go away. Eventually the episode has to be redefined as a problem requiring action. Such actions, in turn, require the reorganization of everyday life. This may occur because of sheer debilitation or because of the disruption engendered by the symptoms. It may occur because the symptoms, especially the blood, are taken to signify extreme danger.

Over the years social and behavioural scientists have written a good deal about the processes whereby symptoms are noticed and acted or not acted upon, and the speed with which actions may follow. David Mechanic is a seminal figure in this regard. Although he subsequently wrote a great deal on the topic his earliest writings seem to be the most succinct. He argued that four elements entered into a social-psychological calculus to shape people's behaviour in the face of symptoms. These four elements were: the frequency with which illness occurs in a given population; the relative familiarity of the symptoms to the average member of the group; the relative predictability of the outcome of the illness; and the amount of threat or loss that is likely to arise as a result of the illness (Mechanic, 1962). The diarrhoea and debilitation that occur in colitis are both frequent and familiar. Blood in the stool is not. Once the symptoms take off into an acute phase, the outcome becomes extremely unpredictable and threat and loss may loom large. This may explain why the respondents acted when and in the way they did.

Zola is another important author who made a specialized study of the early phases of illness. He focused on variables such as psychological distress and concluded that such distress was important in the decision to seek help (Stoeckle et al., 1964; Zola, 1965, 1966). Zola went on to elaborate five triggers which were involved in the decision to seek treatment. These were: interpersonal crises, social interference, sloughing off responsibility to others, perceived threat, and the nature and quality of symptoms. There are elements of these things in the reported behaviour of the subjects. However, the term the subjects would most often use to describe what has happened was 'coping'. They would see their initial encounter with their symptoms as one in which they had to cope with their changed body functioning. This might include going to a doctor, but coping is not analogous to seeking medical help. To get a fuller understanding of the behavioural mechanisms it is necesary to go beyond the work of Mechanic and Zola.

The theory of coping, and in particular that developed by Richard Lazarus, the American psychologist, is highly illuminating in respect of colitis. Lazarus has studied and written about coping over many years. His position may be summarized as follows. All human life gives rise to stresses and strains and from time to time all humans find that such stresses and strains exceed their ability to deal with them. At this point a stimulus exists in the environment which has to be confronted. The way in which a stimulus comes to be defined as stressful is quite complex but can be summarized as the processes of appraisal – primary appraisal and secondary appraisal. Primary appraisal involves an assessment of danger, secondary appraisal involves an assessment of how to deal with that danger. When the individual confronts a stress or strain – a stimulus – the process of primary appraisal determines whether he or she views the stimulus as irrelevant, benign or stressful. If this stimulus is viewed as irrelevant or benign no action need be taken. If, however, something is appraised as stressful, this is because it represents harm or loss, threat (which is anticipated harm or loss) or a challenge. In these cases action has to follow. Secondary appraisal *is* the action and is the coping process. Secondary appraisal is the assessment of what can be done following the primary appraisal. Secondary appraisal is about mastering the condition of harm, threat or challenge, when a routine or automatic response is unavailable. Sometimes coping involves direct action and problem solving, other times it is about palliation, which means finding some way of regulating the emotional distress. Coping can involve seeking information, taking direct action, not doing anything, or internal psychic activity (conscious or unconscious) (Lazarus, 1980; Lazarus and Folkman, 1984a, 1984b; Monat and Lazarus, 1985).

This model is extremely helpful when describing what happens in the case of the onset of colitis. Almost invariably when the symptoms initially appear they are not recognized (appraised) as a disease. Prospective patients do of course observe a deviation from normality in their bowel habit, but the typical response (the primary appraisal) is to define such deviations as irrelevant, benign, or within the range of normal experience. This is not at all unreasonable because diarrhoea and even pain are well within the range of normal experience and as such can be routinely coped with by doing nothing. However, the appearance of blood, in particular, signals the need to revise the individual's initial primary appraisal of irrelevance and harmlessness. The prospective patient will begin to cope with the problems that the diarrhoea or other discomforts are themselves causing, especially the need to maintain normal appearances in the face of embarrassing symptoms.

At the point at which the individual translates self-indicated changes in bodily normality into problems which significantly interfere with desired or required role responsibilities, or at the point at which benign symptoms are reappraised as symbolically highly threatening, for example because of the appearance of blood, seeking help is then deemed to be legitimate.

Seeking help, it was shown, could take a number of forms, either medical, or non-medical or alternative-medical. These constitute direct actions and information-gathering in the secondary appraisal process. Once the person has initiated contact with the medical profession, this sometimes opens up a range of new problems which themselves have to be coped with, in addition to the ongoing symptoms. For some respondents initial contact with their doctors did not only *not* lead to a diagnosis (not in itself clinically unusual) but met with a denial of the problem by the physician. The proto-patients' theory that they have a serious problem is dismissed, and their earlier benign hypothesis is confirmed.

If symptoms remit, this is not a problem. However, symptoms do persist and respondents have to re-engage with their medical advisers. From the point of view of coping, the proto-patients are coping both with their symptoms and with the primary care system. This may involve the sufferer having recourse to 'inappropriate' non-medical or alternative medical treatments, or to direct action to try and educate the medical practitioner.

However, not all of respondents faced this problem and for all of them their physicians eventually recognized the legitimacy of their behaviour in seeking medical help. Diagnoses were made or, more usually, onward referral to appropriate specialist hospital care was made. Diagnosis is highly significant in the coping process because not only does it lead to treatments which may be partly or wholly effective in alleviating the worst aspects of the symptoms, and not only does it provide a legitimation to the patient for having sought out treatment (their coping strategy is justified) but also the disease label provides an explanation of what has been going on for weeks, months or years. Sometimes diagnosis itself may be viewed as a threat, especially where the certainty of diagnosis ends an uncertainty which the patients may have wished to preserve. Sometimes people's lives become bound up in their illness in ways they find psychologically satisfying. For them the threat is to their enjoyment of the sick role. The much more common reaction, however, was for diagnosis to be a positive relief and a positive coping resource in so far as it helped to make sense, in a way that was recognizable to others, of that which had hitherto been rather frightening.

Chapter three

Living with ulcerative colitis

The novelty of changes in bodily functioning sooner or later wears off. Eventually, the person with ulcerative colitis has to settle into a routine with his or her illness and its symptoms. These become facts of life which have to be coped with. Relationships with other people may change as the sufferer alters their daily routine or withdraws from particular social situations. Family life may be affected, as the person with the illness begins to spend an increasing amount of time in the toilet or becomes excessively concerned about his or her diet. Work or school may be disrupted as the individual is forced to take sick leave.

For some people their health shows a dramatic and obvious downturn. They feel ill, they look ill and everyone else recognizes the fact that they have problems. For other people with colitis the symptoms are unpredictable and the spells of good and bad health are cyclical. They do not always look ill, nor do they always feel ill. They may be obliged to, or may want to, carry on as normal, and they may successfully do so for periods of time. Their problem is that they are not unambiguously ill, and dealing with and adjusting to the episodic nature of their problem is the major coping task.

Symptoms

The symptom which tends to become most familiar to the sufferer is the chronic but unpredictable diarrhoea. Diarrhoea and controlling it are prominent features of life. Martha describes this as follows: 'I don't think I was ever really clear of it. When I thought I was feeling quite well, I wasn't really, I was still having to run to the loo several times a day. There was hardly a day went past, but I didn't. I just couldn't sit through things like the telephone ringing, I would have to run to the toilet. I wouldn't really pass anything from the bowel, but you felt the agitation there.' Here Martha is describing the not uncommon symptom of tenesmus. She would run to the toilet, open her bowel but then be unable to defecate. Sometimes she did have diarrhoea, so she could not take the chance and not go to the toilet, for fear of self-soiling. Even when her symptoms were at a low level she still had to organize her life around the toilet.

In some phases of the illness, it may be utterly debilitating. 'You were sometimes just caught slightly short, by the time you'd got there. I was surprised at the frequency. It was much more often than I realized. Some nights you would go to your bed and you'd be absolutely beat, just with running up the stairs and wondering if you would make it', was the way Bernadette described the experience of fatigue and exhaustion. Pauline had similar difficulties. 'At the time I just felt terrible, ill all the time. I wasn't able to do anything towards the end, and I had a sore stomach all the time. I was never getting a night's sleep, I didn't have a full night's sleep in a whole year. I was always coming down to the toilet, and then I just really felt ill and tired all the time.' Pauline was describing another symptomatic feature of colitis, which is that the bowel does not become quiescent during sleep. It continues to be active and the urgent need to go to the toilet can interrupt sleep, as in Pauline's case, over a prolonged period of time.

Weight loss and general ill health are other common problems. 'I couldn't do anything. I didn't have any energy. I felt so pathetic. I found it difficult to believe that anything made you feel quite so low. I just didn't have any energy at all. All I wanted to do was sleep. I could barely eat anything and keep it down. I was down to about six stones by that stage. I was pretty pathetic', said Melanie. In extreme cases, like Maggie's, any semblance of normal life was out of the question: 'Well most of the time I spent in bed. I didn't like being in bed. I tried to come down and I did come down most of the day. But as soon as I got into bed my husband was up. I needed a bed pan, I needed a sick bowl. I went on like this week after week after week, until it was getting that I could hardly lift my hand, even to lift a cup to my mouth, I was so weak. Half the time I wasn't conscious.'

In each of the preceding extracts the sufferer was totally involved in his or her illness. The whole person, or sense of self, was intimately and inextricably bound up with the disease. There was no escape from chronic severe symptoms. These extracts demonstrate that being ill and having a sense of self as an ill person are of course all obvious and natural responses to the disease. However, total involvement in and resignation to the illness are also ways of coping with it. When Lazarus described 'doing nothing' as a means of secondary appraisal, he was describing the type of coping when it is useless or fruitless to try to do anything else. The sufferer's world is turned upside down by the symptoms, which come to dominate every aspect of life. There is very little by way of active resistance that he or she can do. The best way to deal with the illness is to let it take over, albeit temporarily, until a spell of remission begins. What should also be noted about the above extracts is that, with the exception of Maggie, all the other respondents continued in their full-time occupations throughout these periods of debilitation, with only a limited amount of time away from work. However, work performances not frequently became attenuated. As this was realized by the sufferer, and by others, as they had their days off, and as they increasingly missed longer and longer spells of work, the illness began to take them over. Defining themselves as sick, of course, helped to justify the attenuated performance of work and other roles, and eased the difficulties of trying to carry on.

Pain and uncertainty

Pain and uncertainty are aspects of the experience of ulcerative colitis that may be a constant accompaniment of everyday living. Irene describes her pain as follows: 'This pain was constantly there. I used to sit like this, all tensed up, or like this [*she bent forwards folding her arms across her abdomen*]; it was easier to sit like this, to relieve some of the pain. It was always there and although you more or less got immune to it, it also came to the point where it was so bad, that it affected everything else I did.' For some people the pain was episodic rather than chronic. Shena, a factory worker, emphasised this. 'I couldn't move for it. If I got pain, if it hit me, I couldn't move. If I was standing up or maybe walking, I'd have to stop until it went, I was frightened to move.' Georgina's pain had a sudden and unpredictable quality. 'It was terrible. Just a sudden urgency to go to the loo. The cramps in my stomach were like contractions. Then you'd come off and you'd sit for a quarter of an hour and there you were back again. It always seemed worse at night time. It was very very painful.'

The significant part about these extracts is not that each of these subjects experienced pain. What is remarkable is what is absent from these and most other descriptions of the experience of pain in colitis in the interviews. Attempts to relieve pain, particularly by seeking out medical help or using analgesics do not figure in the accounts. What seems to occur is that pain becomes incorporated into people's private view of normal self. They come to see themselves as those for whom pain (acute or chronic) is a way of life and a background feature of all social and other activity. It should also be noted that while the above extracts refer to extreme pain many subjects reported continuous, lower-grade pain as a constant feature of their colitis.

In contrast to the ubiquitousness and the certainty about pain, it was the uncertainty of the cure of the illness and the uncertainty about the diarrhoea which was another dominant feature. As regards the illness itself Shena explains: 'I was in hospital for two months and I really came very good. But it kept coming back. It would go away for a spell, then it would come back. And every time it came back it got worse.' Martin, a railwayman, likewise: 'I could go for long periods with no problems, and then I would get a sudden bout of ulcerative colitis, but in the meantime I would go for months and months, and then bang! back to the beginning again.'

The next extract is from the interview with Christine. She had a cyclical course, although her problems got considerably worse at each successive major attack. In the end the spells of good health were a rarity. 'I used to spend nights down in the lounge. I would give myself prednisolone enemas. I would lay on my side and put the enema in. As soon as it was in, it would just give way and everything would come away out, and I would also vomit. These were the kind of things I went through. I'd wake up another two or three times in the night with the same thing. I wasted away something terrible at times. Then I'd spend another eight or nine weeks in hospital, slowly getting back to normal.' An extract from Melanie's interview shows that the cyclical course can itself be very rapid. 'I came home for a week's holiday and I didn't feel particularly well, went away for a few days and felt dreadful, was in bed. I couldn't eat anything, I couldn't keep anything down, I couldn't keep anything in. I went on to steroids. That cleared it up and I was fine by the beginning of September. Mid-way through October I didn't feel very well again. I felt bad for about two weeks. Went back to hospital and more steroids, and then I haemorrhaged badly.'

In each of these cases the main theme is uncertainty. The uncertainty attaches to the unpredictable course of remission and exacerbation. In each case, at periods of exacerbation the illness got worse. The unpredictability itself represented a threat. Likewise the limitations which the symptoms impose also represent a threat. In Martin's case his coping mechanism was to carry on as normal and, as he revealed elsewhere, to try to resist his doctor's attempts to get him to consider surgery. In both Christine and Melanie's cases attempts were made to carry on as normal in the face of increasingly debilitating symptoms.

Loss of control and diet

In some cases ulcerative colitis is an invisible illness. Someone ignorant of a colitic's diagnosis or history, may not become aware of his or her condition simply by observing the sufferer's appearance. Other people with colitis, however, will be thin and pale, wasted and emaciated. Whatever they look like, their social behaviour may appear to be odd. The person with colitis is likely very suddenly to break off conversations, meals, indeed any social interaction, in order to go to the toilet. One of the problems someone with colitis faces in these circumstances will be the attempt to preserve some semblance of normality when the symptoms are intrusive. This is not always easy because there are a number of things relating to symptom manifestation which may undermine competent presentation of self. One of these is diet.

For someone with colitis eating and drinking can be associated in a very immediate way with the symptoms of the illness. As soon as they consume food or drink they may need to open their bowel. Bernadette explained: 'As soon as you ate something, before you virtually finished your meal, anything you seemed to put in your mouth just seemed to trigger off this diarrhoea and you were running.' And Tom, a joiner, said, 'If I had a cold drink, I had this sensation I had to go to the toilet. When I went to the toilet there was nothing. And when you thought, that's that and went back and took another drink it was the same. I would walk into a place and maybe go to the toilet twelve or fourteen times.'

The significance of this is in people's private view of themselves; they are constantly aware of the possibility that their food and liquid intake might trigger an attack, and they are constantly on the look-out for toilets. The significance also relates to the way others respond to this behaviour; the kinds of social labels or social identities which become attached to this type of conduct may be important. Getting up suddenly from the dinner table at home in the company of close family, may be one thing; to do so in other contexts such as a formal dinner, or during a meeting may draw unwanted attention to the behaviour. Furthermore, the widespread ritual and culturally significant nature of food and drink consumption (Christmas dinners, wedding breakfasts, formal banquets) makes the breaking of social convention by making frequent exits to the toilet something which has to be coped with. The behaviour may well pass without comment, but a form of rule breaking it is none the less.

The difficulty for the person with colitis is that his or her attempt to present a relatively normal self to others is continually being threatened, because of the inherently unstable nature of the condition. This means that impression management is always precarious. The abrupt termination of interaction shatters the illusion upon which much social behaviour (especially intimate social contact) is based, that is, that the participants are focused on the matter in hand. Suddenly dashing off to the toilet suggests that the colitic has more pressing matters on his or her mind and that his or her attention is elsewhere.

Avoidance of social situations, such as public eating and drinking, or elaborate strategies to control food intake are therefore, unsurprisingly, reported by many respondents. Norah said, 'Many things upset it: pastry, fatty things, bran, oatcakes, bread, chips, fried fish, fried food, curries, spicy food, things with currants, things with sultanas, fruit. So I ate soup, chicken, white meat, mince and potatoes, shepherd's pie and poached white fish. It was so boring. But I kept reasonably well. If I went and ate any of the foods I wasn't supposed to eat, that would aggravate it, and everything would be worse.' Rhona ate 'Angel Delight and very soft food'. Marjorie drank only Coca Cola, and Martha avoided vegetables. Each respondent found his or her own way of handling their diet. Some would take risks in spite of the known consequences. Gwen, for example, said 'I used to have curry and would still have curry. I would suffer for two days, but it didn't stop me having it.'

The respondents reported acquiring knowledge, on a trial and error basis, about their colitis and their diet. This is not an unreasonable thing to do and suggests a realistic recognition of the limitations the disease places upon self. Theirs is an acknowledgement of themselves as ill. This does not preclude risk-taking in pursuit of the pleasure of a particular favourite food, but the consequences of such indiscretions also become part of self.

Loss of control linked directly to diet, or more general loss of control, was a theme much discussed in the interviews. Georgina said, 'I used to find that I didn't have any confidence to go out anywhere, because I was frightened. All of a sudden you'd be sitting and you'd need to go.' Martha resorted to counting her visits to the toilet. 'It wasn't under control. I was keeping a chart; twenty-two, twenty-three times a day I was in the loo.' Constant visits to the toilet or the constant worry that such visits might be imminent serve to undermine adult identity. In particular the notion that most other adults can, and should, control their bowels, is thrown open to very public doubt. Loss of control represents the potential, or anticipated potential, for humiliation and disgrace attendant upon the spoiled interaction. In some cases, face is saved simply by withdrawal; people stop going to the places where such public humiliation might occur. Others carry on resolutely (more of which below). In the context of their public identities people with colitis who do not adopt the sick role need to present to the external world a version of self which others identify as normal. Where things go wrong, the reaction may be embarrassment, itself a stress to be coped with. Willie, a craftsman, said, 'I was sore with myself, embarrassed with having to run home after a night out with my wife. Even if I only had two or three pints, I'd have to leave her at the top of the road to run home.'

Georgina, Martha and Willie all refer to threats to being taken seriously as adults. Adult men and women, whatever their social class, whatever their other social roles, are obviously adults who, in western culture, do not defecate uncontrollably in public. It is one of the basic distinguishing features of adulthood, as against infancy, early childhood and old age that control of the anal sphincter is a taken-for-granted accomplishment. The loss of that control is not only at odds with being an adult, it also suggests flawed moral character.

Relationships

Loss of control affects and threatens relationships with other people, at home, at work and in leisure time. Relatives and friends will become drawn into the illness in various ways. Shena said, 'My husband is the only serious boyfriend I ever had, and really it's amazing. He'd take me home on a date and we're standing having a necking session, and I'd have to go away to the toilet. He was really good back up, he was really good.' Shena's boyfriend adjusted to Shena's need to keep going to the toilet and loved her anyway. Others were much less fortunate. Jane, a former barmaid said, for example, 'I'd had to stay in the house all the time, I was virtually a prisoner. I couldn't go out because everywhere I went I had to make sure there was a toilet. When I tried to explain to the boyfriend, he just couldn't understand. We split up eventually.' Irene tried to exclude her boyfriend from her experience 'It disrupted our relationship at times, and I would just say, "Look, I feel awful, I'm in a bad mood, a foul temper, I feel ill, tired, I don't want to see you."'

The point to note is that while the disease disrupts the normal course of the relationship, different consequences follow from this. In Irene's case the symptoms disrupted the relationship and she coped by withdrawing temporarily from it and explaining her withdrawal in terms of her being a sick person. The coping mechanism is the creation of the sick identity in which it is taken for granted that ordinary relationships may legitimately be discontinued because of the illness. Shena drew her boyfriend into her coping strategy. Together they effectively carried on as normally as they could, while accommodating to the disease's symptoms. They did it together. In Jane's case the boyfriend did not want to know and he was the prime mover in terminating his involvement in the relationship.

Family life can be affected by the disease. Whether the sufferer is a child, a young person living at home, or someone living independently of parents, with or without their own spouse and children, significantly affects the extent to which the family is involved. Also important is the extent to which the family unit bands together to deal with the illness.

For people who had already attained independence from their parents economically, domestically or simply by virtue of their age, there appeared to be a tendency to try and minimize the extent to which parents were involved in the management of the illness. In particular adult sons and daughters seemed to be at pains to conceal the true extent of their symptoms. The independence already enjoyed by these respondents allowed them to try to present themselves to their parents as normal adult sons or daughters untarnished by disease. Tracy, a clerk, explained, 'I was living in my flat, on my own, and the most important person in my life was that person I was having a relationship with. I told him everything because he was my support and comfort. I told less to my family because my family worry. I told them the minimum.'

In the next extract Donna, who was a student living at home when her illness began, shows how together she and her family controlled the flow of information about the illness. They colluded together to show nothing was wrong even though her behaviour must have been noted as odd. 'My parents were really the sort who didn't mention that sort of thing. I mean they would be aware, but they wouldn't mention it. Breakfast time was the worst time. I mean I would eat my breakfast and knew I would be doubled up.' Bill, a clerk, never even mentioned his problem to the ageing mother and father with whom he lived. 'I didn't say any thing when I first got the trouble, it was only a couple of years later that I said anything. I didn't want to.'

For persons who have family responsibilities themselves, the colitis can cause problems which are simply not manageable by information control. Caroline, a newly-wed housewife when her disease started, had to move back to her mother's house. 'I just had a year of total diarrhoea, and pain, I had to stay with my mother. We didn't have a bath, so I moved in with my mother.' Christine, who had a young family, found life extremely difficult. 'I could never go out normally and take the kids out. I could never take her far in the pram because I had no energy and I couldn't go far without being near a toilet. It tells on the kids. It didn't tell on the little one, but it did on the other two. And my husband had to suffer too. He had to come home some nights to an empty house if the kids were staying at my mother's.' Joyce, a local government worker, fared rather better. 'They've all grown up with me being like that and they have all worked in with it. I can't honestly remember any difficulty with any of them really. They grew up with me being like this, and Jean the oldest one, she was always good at doing things, and doing the shopping and the housework.'

These extracts are from subjects who were young adults at the time of the onset. In contrast Peter, a civil servant, had an onset in early middle age when he himself had a growing family. He and his wife and children consciously disregarded the illness and colluded together to do so. 'Oh it didn't affect the family because they all had their own bedrooms. They accepted it. They didn't know much about it, of course, I just went on. They knew I had it, but I tried to live a life that would make it as quiet as possible. I would attend to it, just as if it were a normal illness.' Bernadette's son was 'rather oblivious to the whole thing. I mean his mother had diarrhoea again. But I didn't think he was even really concerned about it. I don't think he was very aware of it. It was an inconvenience. If they were in the loo, and I had to get in there, and they had to come out. That's where they suffered more than anything, because they weren't really aware of how bad it was.'

For both Peter and Bernadette, their identities as father or mother were intact but as father- or mother-with-an-illness, which was played down and accommodated to, in order to preserve the broader patterns of family life. Joyce's family helped and Christine's family suffered, while Caroline reassumed the role of daughter living at home.

Outside the family many respondents continued working while their disease progressed and thus held on to the identity of employee or worker. In some cases special circumstances helped; Willie, for example, said, 'I didn't lose a lot of days off work because I didn't work for a firm, I was on my own, I was my own boss so I could nip off to the loo and if I was feeling really lousy I could just knock off and go home.' Others were less fortunate and just had to take time off and lose money as a consequence. This happened to Shena, for example: 'I was working in a factory at the time and I was off my work a lot.'

In order to continue working, some degree of flexibility is required, or support from employers is needed. The attempt to maintain as normal a life as possible can be helped by sympathetic employers and workmates. Workmates, employers or family members – or all three – have to do something to help.

Joyce's case illustrates the point. 'I very seldom lost any time off my work. I didn't realize I looked as bad as I did. It was only afterwards when people told me. And going to work, we had to stop along the road to go to the loo somewhere, but very seldom did I allow it to interfere. And when we went out, my husband and our friends were all looking and checking where the loos were, because I mean, that was the way, the life we had to lead.' Joyce's normality was bolstered by the fact that her workmates did not tell her how ill she looked, by the fact that her husband stopped the car at least once every day on the way to work so she could go to the toilet (it was a fifteen-minute drive), and by the fact that her close friends would scan the environment for toilets wherever they went. She was someone who was sick and therefore enjoyed special privileges but she acted as normally as possible.

Sometimes people confront organizations or individuals who will not be flexible. Gloria for example, worked in a hospital. 'I was talking to somebody and went into the sluice for something, and that was it. It just came from me. It was torture. And sister took one look at me, and my uniform was saturated: it was very embarrassing for me. She told me to go home. But I said I would just change and get on with my work. But she sent me home anyway. I was back the next day, but I was caught out.'

Gloria's story is interesting because it shows a workmate refusing to go along with an obviously sick person's attempt to act normally. In this instance the ward sister treated the episode as a medical one rather than colluding with Gloria to hide the problem. Gloria was able to get back to work the next day. The sanctions imposed on her were temporary. However, some respondents had to face inflexible bureaucratic and legal rules which were non-negotiable. Mike had to attend a medical to join the prison service: 'I was not in the best of health, but never said anything about it at the time, and I got the next interview. By the time they offered me the job I'd been diagnosed as having colitis. So I then wrote and told them. They then wanted a report from the doctor. They wrote back to say that they were sorry but on the basis of their medical officer's report they could not appoint me.'

The prison service defined Mike as sick. Whatever attempts he may have made to present a normal self was denied by the bureaucratic processes of recruitment. The contrast between Gloria's and Mike's cases demonstrates that some identities are negotiable and others are not. Gloria's story shows that a veneer of normality can be maintained so long as other people engage in behaviours which dovetail with those of the patient. The moment others fail to do this then the strategy falls apart.

Fighting back and carrying on regardless

Home and work provide familiar surroundings for most people; the great thing about a familiar environment, from the point of view of someone with colitis, is that it provides not just sanctuary from the outside world, but also safe and easy access to toilets. When a person is removed from a safe and familiar environment, when travelling for example, the lack of toilet facilities is very threatening. The strategies most commonly adopted in the face of this are the restriction of travel, elaborate planning of journeys in such a way that toilets are available, planning the time of journeys to avoid periods when the bowel might be active, and the acquisition of elaborate knowledge of the whereabouts of toilets.

Gwen described her problems. 'I wouldn't go anywhere far. I would venture down to the shops. We did go to my mother-in-law's but always stopped at the same place on the way. I could never relax, I was always worried until I got to the door.' Caroline found shopping a problem: 'I didn't enjoy shopping or anything. I was always wanting to be near a toilet. We couldn't plan anything, I'd never know if I'd be able to.' Georgina tried taking a foreign holiday. 'I always got this feeling. I used to wander around saying "Oh God, what if I have to go to the toilet?" That's what you wonder all the time, and then dying to turn back to the hotel to use the loo, and then sit there for ages because you felt safe.' Nevertheless, people with colitis do try to keep going in spite of the threat which leaving home presents.

For some respondents the disease was something which had to be actively resisted and fought back against. Resisting the illness does not involve pretending that there is no illness, so much as recognizing the limits or problems that the disease presents and challenging those problems. Whatever activities are involved, such as continuing to work, or fulfilling other role responsibilities, the person is able to think of himself or herself as getting back at, rather than submitting to the illness. Andrew said, 'You start getting a wee bit annoyed and aggressive with yourself and you say, "God, I'll try and beat this at all costs". You find you go through the whole spectrum of emotions. As long as you have the disease you've got to find some sort of acceptance in your mind.'

For Harry the fighting spirit manifested itself in his struggle to keep working. 'I got to the stage where on virtually a daily basis I couldn't walk down the road to go to work. At that time I worked in Dumbarton. It was only four or five hundred yards from where I lived. I had to wear paper underpants and sanitary towels amongst them.' Benny, a seaman, fought back in very practical ways. 'I kept a note of just how often I was actually having to run to the toilet. I think it was anything between fifteen and twenty times. I'd go to bed, think "Great, I can get some sleep" and about an hour later, bang, that was it. I always took a change of underwear with me, knowing that where we would be would have a toilet. You couldn't be more than about five minutes from the toilet.'

Fighting back or resisting involves practical coping to meet difficulties. This is slightly different from another common reaction, which can be described as 'carrying on regardless'. This involves ignoring the difficulties. Martha explained: 'Sometimes it was just the difficulty of managing to get out to work. They'd all be sitting in the car, and I'd be running into the house again, to go to the loo. It was ridiculous. I really wasn't away from work ill. I just managed to keep going. And I think this is where I felt, well it can't be that bad because I'm coping. I'm managing. So when I would go up for visits to the hospital, I'd say "Fine, fine, fine, everything's fine." As long as I was managing to get into work and get home again I was fine.' Martha did non-manual work; Georgina worked in a factory, so her problems were slightly different. 'I'd stand and say to myself, "Oh God, please don't let me have to run to the loo, please don't let me." I mean a woman's factory, full of women in the toilets all the time. Sure as fate when I used to get myself all tensed up that's when it would start. And then I used to say to myself "Maybe if I didn't eat anything at lunchtime that'll help." I used to think if I didn't put anything in my stomach there would be nothing to come through, but it doesn't work like that.'

Tracy also found her work life dominated by the toilet. 'If you were quite well you could manage to go to the loo once an hour. But if you were really bad you'd be back up again, and you were worn out, completely worn out before half a day had gone. I was working at that time too . . . my boss and the men in the office just accepted the fact that I was in the loo.'

The attempt to keep going in the face of these kinds of problems is a form of active coping. The greater the attempt to carry on as normal the greater the tension for self. Fiona, a clerk, explained. 'It's something about us folk. We sort of carry on regardless. I remember going out to work, I really couldn't work. But I went anyway because I wasn't incapable of work. You know the feeling. You aren't in a state of total collapse. So I kept going to work.' And Norah, 'When it was worse, I would get to the point where I still would not admit that I was ill, and I would still try to go out. I didn't want to admit that I was ill, and that this was going to destroy or mix up my plans. So I just went on.'

Fighting back and carrying on regardless are not individual behaviours. They are social behaviours which involve other people. Joyce said, 'I thought, "Damn, it's not going to beat me. I'll beat it." And we generally went on holiday with six or eight of us, so there was no way I was going to be the one to call off, just because of ulcerative colitis. The year before we went to Ilfracombe because I just couldn't possibly go abroad.'

Joyce's comment encapsulates the ideas both of involving other people and of limiting social activity. Six to eight people had to change their usual holiday arrangements of having a holiday in Spain to having a holiday in Devon. Joyce made a realistic, or what she took to be a realistic, assessment of the risk associated with going abroad. She stated a determination to appear normal. She would not cancel her holiday and she tried to minimize the possibly disruptive effects of her symptoms by staying both in the orbit of the NHS and a familiar sanitary system.

The price exacted for Joyce being able to 'beat it' was that others had to alter their behaviour. In effect she was able to carry on as normal while others changed in ways which they may not have thought desirable. Other respondents behaved in the same way, although ostensibly involving fewer people. Gwen, for example, said, 'I must admit that my husband was very good. He understood because he saw what it was like. But I felt with friends, they didn't, they couldn't understand why I was so worried about going out anywhere. If we went away with friends I felt I was holding them back. I never spoke to many people about it. Just close friends. They were the only ones that knew.' It was her husband, however, whose life was transformed by the illness. He altered his working and holiday arrangements in order to allow Gwen to live as full and active life as possible.

Nevertheless, trying to carry on regardless can produce situations of real threat. Mary said, 'I was going down to visit a friend in Trowbridge in Wiltshire, and I remember thinking "What if I get diarrhoea while I'm staying with her?" ' Shena, likewise, said, 'I used to be terrified of going to people's houses. It was okay going to friends because they understood, we made a joke of it, but you can only take it so far.' Shena's point is that there is a limit beyond which special dispensations or allowances will not be provided by other people to sustain the pretence or the appearance of carrying on regardless. Rhona's comment in her next extract suggests that she reached that point and withdrew from social contact as a consequence. 'Your friends are sympathetic up to a point, but they don't want you going out with them. You could be taken ill and they don't want to worry about you all night. I didn't want to be "Rhona who is ill."'

For some people the issue ceased to be a social or a psychological one when their symptoms simply overwhelmed them, and when carrying on regardless did not work. Julie explained it thus: 'Things got very bad. It was making me late for work. I'd be up most of the night, I was tired. I'd fly in and out of the loo in the morning. I'd go out of the door to go to work and decide that I had to come back again to go to the loo. I thought I must go to work, but I had to keep going to the loo. Often that would happen three or four times. I'd be out in my car and thinking I'll have to go back in again. There were the concerts I used to go to. You don't want to be embarrassed, or embarrass your friends by getting up half-way through. So I simply opted out. More often than not I would make my way out to these things, and on my way there, I would decide I'd better not and turn back. I've seen me do that many times.'

In this and other examples like it, withdrawal is not a permanent retreat to being an invalid. It is a temporary withdrawal contingent upon circumstances. There are certain circumstances, attending a public concert, or trying to go to work, where other people simply cannot help in glossing things over. Routine negotiation, turning a blind eye or ignoring, making a joke, or other people simply easing the person through their difficulty are either impossible or inappropriate. The subject's illness and its symptoms provide a public identity which transcend all attempts to carry on regardless. In these circumstances withdrawal is a highly rational behaviour.

Making sense of it all

Human beings are engaged constantly in a process of making sense of the world around them. This is particularly so if something in the environment seems odd, alarming, or out of the ordinary. A major illness and all the changes which follow from that illness require explanation. People are compelled by circumstances to try and make sense of what is happening to them.

Some of the subjects wanted to understand the cause of their illness. Georgina and her family put it down to diet. 'They just thought that I had one of these things that's like an upset stomach. I always thought it would get better. I always thought it was like an allergy. Maybe if they found what I was eating it would go away.' Georgina identified what she took to be a definite cause and for a while at least, experimented with this idea by trying out different kinds of diets in the expectation of some improvement. For other people in the study the very close scrutiny of their own signs and symptoms allowed them to discover an explanation. Gwen said, 'When I worked it was better than when I didn't. It's possible that not having anything to occupy my mind made me worry more, and when you work it takes your mind off it.' Mary used some knowledge of basic biology to impute a cause. 'My mind said worm infestations. I was absolutely terrified to go and see a doctor.'

One thing many of the respondents were aware of was the possible psychological or psychosomatic aetiology of ulcerative colitis. Some patients rejected such a view. Shena, for example, was told by her GP that the death of her father may have been a trigger which started off her illness. She did not believe this. Peter's doctor kept seeking out some underlying worries which Peter allegedly had. 'I had no sorts of worries at all. At least I thought I didn't have anything to worry about. I was told I was worrying about something, but I don't know what I was worrying about. The surgeon would say "You must be worried about something." And I said, "Nothing at all." ' Other respondents mentioned stress, anxiety and mood. What was notable about these responses was that while many people showed some awareness of the psychological cum psychosomatic arguments about colitis, none of them thought them tenable. It might well be, he argued, that they needed to reject the psychological type of explanation because it would be inherently more threatening than one based upon physical or physiological origins. It is as if to admit to the possibility of a psychological aetiology is tantamount to admitting there is something wrong with one's mind. The explanation may, however, be simpler than this, because few physicians and still fewer surgeons who treated these respondents and were thus a major source of information for them, seemed to have much time for psychodynamic types of explanation.

The ways in which the subjects in this study tried to explain and account for what had happened to them and what was happening to them, drew upon a variety of sources: their direct experiences, information they received from medical practitioners, their previous experiences, and various pre-existing knowledge, attitudes and beliefs. They drew upon common-sense ideas about the nature of cause and effect and about diseases. Such ideas helped to explain the predicament they found themselves in. Equally their understanding of the ways other people responded to them was made the more meaningful by these ideas. Their disease and its symptoms are omnipresent either actually or in the sense of being likely to break through at any moment. Symptoms become an integral part of everyday life. Some are appraised as being beyond self-control (pain particularly), whereas the suddenness of defecation has to be dealt with and cannot be ignored. The routine uncertainty of the bowel motion requires detailed scanning of the environment and the planning of activities in ways in which uncertainty might be minimized. Nevertheless, planning and scanning the environment cannot be done to the exclusion of everything else because competent role performance in other spheres of life is demanded. Thus people try to carry on anyway and fight back, and they have to bring into their struggle other people who can help in collusion, pretence and the creation of the illusion of normality. It is a social activity requiring much hard work to sustain it.

Conclusion

Many writers have considered the kinds of problems with which the person with colitis has to deal from a social and psychological point of view in respect of other chronic illnesses. The striking thing about many such studies is that while the symptoms of rheumatoid arthritis, Parkinson's disease, or diabetes, for example, are clearly different from those of colitis, in many ways the problems posed by such illnesses have a quality which cuts across particular medical diagnosis and is common to them all. The disruption occasioned by chronic illness has been very sensitively documented from a sociological point of view by Bury (1982), while Williams (1984) has highlighted (in the case of rheumatoid arthritis), just how important the attempts to make sense of what is happening in chronic illness really are. That people develop strategies for dealing with their chronic illness is a familiar theme in the sociological literature. Wiener (1975), for example, identified particular strategies which sufferers with rheumatoid arthritis develop in order to tolerate the uncertainty produced by that disease. Many of the things she reported mirror closely the activities noted in this chapter. She observed that her subjects had a psychological strategy of hope, they concealed disability and pain, they tried to keep up with normal activities, they paced themselves, they recognized the limits placed on themselves and they organized their lives accordingly. They also developed lowered expectations and they would elicit help from others who became drawn into the whole process. This echoes a still earlier study of polio victims by Davis (1963) who focused on strategies to deal with that illness. More recently Pinder (1990) provides illuminating data about the constant struggle that Parkinson's disease sufferers and their families are involved in, in order to hold on to any sense of normality.

The work of Strauss and his collaborators (1984) strikes a particular chord with the problems that people with ulcerative colitis have to live with (unsurprisingly, given that colitis is used in that book as one of the examples). Strauss argues that chronic illnesses are characterized by uncertainty in prognosis, treatment (sometimes) and cause (being often episodic). They are deeply intrusive into everyday routines and require great efforts in dealing with pain, discomfort, restricted activity and quality of functioning. The responses tend to be strategic.

Strauss has argued that the controlling of symptoms requires the sufferer to have heightened bodily awareness. Life-styles may need to be reshaped and other people have to be drawn into a process of hiding, minimizing, excusing or disclaiming the illness at the points at which symptoms became intrusive. Both doing these things, and learning to do them, are characterized by sheer hard work and effort. Seeking out information is a typical strategy, according to Strauss, as is withdrawal from social interaction because of actual or potential embarrassment. One of the most fundamental ways of dealing with chronic illness, according to Strauss, is normalizing. Depending on the degree of intrusiveness of the symptoms, keeping things as normal as possible can require enormous effort. Even when working well, there is always an uneasy equilibrium, with the potential for the breakdown of such strategies being ever present.

In a subsequent paper Strauss, with Corbin, has argued that in addition to the physical and emotional work demanded by chronic illness, the sufferer must also fit his or her experiences of illness into the pattern of normal life, must arrive at some degree of understanding and acceptance of the biographical consequences of actual or potential failures, live with the limitations in performance and must rethink the future (Corbin and Strauss, 1987).

All of this writing and much else besides (see, for example, Fagerhaugh, 1973; Reif, 1973a; 1973b; Locker, 1983; Charmaz, 1987; Peyrot *et al.*, 1987; Kelleher, 1988; Pinder, 1988), suggest close parallels across a range of chronic ailments, and that, from a social and psychological point of view, the differences between chronic illnesses are more a matter of emphasis than a matter of physiology, aetiology or any other conventional medical organizing concept.

To bring this chapter to a conclusion the ideas of self and identity will be developed a little more systematically, together with the theory of coping explored in the previous chapter. These ideas will provide the building blocks for the conclusion of the book. At its simplest the term 'self' refers to the inner and private view an individual has of him- or herself, while identity is the public view which others have of that person. Self and identity may be incongruous: the way an individual imagines him- or herself to be, may be distinctly at variance with the way others see that person. The individual may entertain the notion that he or she is young, witty and charming while others may see someone dull, ageing and boring. The relationship between self and identity may be thought of as one of a process of negotiation between individuals. As an individual sets out to present a particular version of self to the world, other people will engage with that person more or less in line with the presentation of self. Selves are presented and then legitimated by others, more or less.

The concept of self has a long and distinguished philosophical and scientific pedigree (Stryker, 1981). Self is defined as an inner and private phenomenon, unique to an individual, unknowable directly to others and which also has a sense of itself. Humans possess a capacity to imagine themselves in the same way that they can see and imagine any other object in the universe. In so doing people are trying to imagine how they appear to others (James, 1968; Cooley, 1981: 171; Mead, 1981: 175-6). Being able to imagine ourselves as others might see us is necessary for rational conduct (Mead, 1934:

138). Self is subjective; it is about our sense of who and what we are, it helps locate us in the world we live; that is, we are someone with particular characteristics, feelings and loyalties. Self is, therefore, an imaginative view of ego. It is essential for psychological functioning and it develops and changes with experience (Kuhn, 1964; McCall and Simmons, 1966; Gergen, 1971; Ball, 1972; Field, 1974; Burke, 1980; Rosenberg, 1981).

Identity is about social relationships. In any social arrangement people occupy positions, statuses and roles. These are the markers by which self is identified by other people. Identity establishes what and where the person is in the social structure. Certain identities are more or less fixed and unchangeable, such as age, gender or race; other identities may change or be the product of social behaviour. Selves are offered and presented and they then may be acknowledged or agreed upon, at which point an identity is established. Identity is related to appearance because roles and statuses are indicated by appearances, badges of office and other signifiers. Particular identities can have a greater or lesser importance at different times (Stone, 1962; Stryker, 1968; Gergen, 1971; Burke, 1980; Rosenberg, 1981; May and Kelly, 1982; Weigart et al., 1986). Identity then is a label imposed by others on self.

Using the concepts of self and identity it is possible to outline the key issues of the experience of colitis. People who have colitis engage in certain kinds of behaviour in the face of their illness. Some of these relate directly to the physical experience of symptoms which become an important part of the person's concept of self, with their importance for self varying as the symptoms come and go. The threats which the symptoms present arise not just from pain, discomfort or even debilitation, but also from their potential to affect identity – the way others define the person. Symptoms have to be incorporated into everyday life, they become a constant feature of self because of their ubiquitous accompaniment to everyday living. Symptoms may indeed become a completely integrated aspect of self because they are what life is all about.

In the face of this, self may have to submit to the illness, but for the most part the subjects of this study reported attempting not just to learn to live with their illness but also to carry on as normal. They tried to present to the external world a view of themselves as ordinary people. Denial, and withdrawal, may be the adjuncts to this, but the unpredictability of bowel function cannot itself be controlled by psychological defence mechanisms, wishful thinking or play-acting. In order to deal with symptoms, subjects develop other strategies such as constantly scanning the environment for escape routes, for toilets and for developing, to a high degree, an awareness of appropriate exit lines (physical and verbal). That awareness also involves habitual planning of activities in order to facilitate scanning and to allow normal functioning. Thus their private selves have to incorporate both the notion of normality and the fact that in order to maintain that normality they have to behave in ways which, on the face of it, are highly odd.

People with colitis face a tension between the demands made upon them by their illness and hence on their selves, and the demands made upon them by normal role obligations, their identities. Their ability to maintain normal role obligations, or their abject failure to do so, will in turn affect self. The tension is marked by the fact that for much of the time, and in many social circumstances, they may attempt to keep concealed the nature of their illness and the compelling nature of the demands of the illness may be shared by only a handful of intimates.

It was noted that in the face of their symptoms and by virtue of the attempt to maintain a veneer of normality through particular presentations of self, many people described their behaviour as 'carrying on regardless' or a similar phrase. However, 'carrying on regardless' is not an activity without costs. It was stressful; sometimes it did not work (and identities were discredited) and sometimes withdrawal was the only way to preserve identity. For other subjects the illness represents a challenge to be fought back against. The distinction between 'carrying on' and 'fighting back' is a fine one; carrying on involves ignoring the symptoms and hence minimizing their salience for self, while fighting back involves incorporating the limitations and problems caused by the symptoms into self and responding accordingly.

In terms of interpersonal relationships during illness two rather different issues arose. With people who are not privy to the 'true' health status of the person, and hence where a normal identity is possible, then the efforts of self are directed towards preserving normality in interaction. The secrecy of the illness and the maintenance of that secrecy means that strangers and people who do not know are not involved in legitimating anything other than the apparently normal version of self. However, this is usually difficult to achieve alone and a group of *cognoscenti* are drawn into the management of the illness in order that a successful, or at least an integrated life beyond the immediate family, can be achieved. The identity which is created with the close-knit kith and kin is that of normal – but ill. The person with colitis is more or less openly acknowledged in the family as someone who is normal, but who has a set of associated illness characteristics which have to be managed.

Various collusive routines were developed, it was noted, to achieve this, including controlling information, and deliberate disregard for, or misinterpretation of, public manifestation of symptoms or their behavioural sequelae. Close intimates not infrequently have to alter their behaviour to maintain the 'normal' identity for the person who is ill. It was also noted that elaborate collusive routines sometimes fail because either a non-intimate fails to collude or a point is reached when collusive practices are deemed inappropriate by self or others.

Chapter four

Having the operation

For many people with colitis there comes a time when the possibility of surgery has to be confronted. A medical practitioner may indicate that because of the state of the patient's health, or because of the life-threatening nature of the illness, surgery is required. For some people such an announcement of medical opinion may be the first time they learn that their disease requires an operation. For the majority, however, when the recommendation for surgery is made, there has already been a period of time during which they have become, or have been made aware of, that possibility. At whatever point the patient learns of the prospect of surgery, a new identity as prospective surgical case needs to be defined. If surgery is a distant possibility the salience of such an identity may be very limited. If, on the other hand, surgery is urgently required, it will be likely to have much greater immediacy for the patient. The degree to which the sense of self is concordant with the identity is critical in understanding the ambivalence shown by many people towards the prospect of surgery.

'I don't want an operation'

Some people expressed great surprise when the operation was first mentioned to them, this in spite of the fact that several had been attending surgical out-patient clinics over many months. Georgina, for example, said, 'My family thought like me that it wasn't serious. Nobody ever mentioned the word operation. So when it came to having an ileostomy they were as shattered as me. They just thought I had an upset stomach.' Tracy made much the same point. 'They never explained to me what it was. I never asked. Maybe that was pretty stupid of me. But I thought it was something you got tablets for or whatever, and you got cured. I never realized that I would have to have an operation.'

The first, and for some subjects, continuing response to the prospect of surgery, was to resist it. Gwen tried not to think about it. 'I just blocked it out. I just didn't want to know. I just couldn't picture it at all. All I knew was that you would have a bag, I just didn't want to know.' In contrast, Andrew sought out as much information as he could in order to try to prove the doctors wrong. He experimented with a range of remedies and was scathing about his medical advisers. 'I wanted to be absolutely sure in my own mind, that I'd tried everything to avoid surgery, because I didn't want it. I don't really think it right that a person has to get that done to them to cure a disease. I believe it should be possible that it can be cured without surgery. I considered surgery the worst possible scenario, having a bag for the rest of your life. By the time it came for me to say "Yes, okay, I'll go through with this operation", I'd really more or less exhausted all my possibilities.'

Some of the subjects developed various subterfuges to put surgery off. Bernadette, for example, said, 'Two days after we came back from our holiday there was a bed for me in the ward. I said, "I've just come back from my holidays, I've got all my washing and ironing to do", and all the excuses came trotting out. I asked what would happen if I didn't come in and was told I would go to the back of the list. She said, "I really think you should come" and I said, "Yes, I know I should come, I'm playing for time here, obviously I'm going to come in but I'm just making excuses." '

Others described resisting up till late in the eleventh hour before the operation. Rhona said, 'I was totally irrational by the time I went in that morning, I was ready to phone up and tell them to forget it. Nobody talked to me about it. I knew what to expect post-operatively because I'd read it, but I didn't know about being catheterized the night before. They came and persuaded me to have the catheter and I think that really brought it home what I was having done, because up until that time I thought I could change my mind at any moment.'

Another subject who refused to acknowledge that she was a prospective surgical case, even after she had been admitted to hospital for the operation, was Marjorie. She claimed that she thought she was going into hospital for tests. 'I got an appointment to go in on Sunday, went in and said, "When am I getting these tests, by the way?" They said, "What tests? You're getting operated on on Tuesday." So there was no going back.'

The resistance to surgery described here may be thought of as an attempt by respondents to maintain the integrity of their 'self' even though such attempts fly in the face of what is going on around them and the identity bestowed upon them by the hospital. Their symptoms are severe and they are in hospital and facing operation, and yet they are behaving in ways which are quite incongruous with their medical and social situation. Their resistance involves such things as intra-psychic blocking, information-seeking, scepticism and disbelief.

In spite of its incongruousness, it is probably inaccurate to describe these behaviours as oddball or bizarre. It certainly might appear to be strange to claim to be in hospital for tests when one is in hospital for major surgery. However, what these types of reactions represent is that most of the subjects found it very difficult to accept the need for surgery. A doctor's recommendation for surgery does not result in automatic acceptance and compliance, especially in such a procedure as this.

In the next extracts the focus is on the transition process. Tracy explained, 'I had been in hospital four days and they said I needed an operation. I felt they could do anything to me, but I didn't want a bag. Then the doctor said, "It'll be fine when you get your bag." Maybe it was a good thing in a way, because if I'd had time to think about it, it might have been a different reaction, but I just felt numb to it.' Tracy had been ill for some time without any knowledge of the possibility of surgery. Her disease then took a turn for the worse. Then, and only then, did she become aware that she would have to have an operation. The transition from someone with a 'sore stomach' to someone needing an urgent major operation was swift. She herself hardly seemed to have had time to take it in. She obviously saw this as helpful with regard to her coping.

For other patients the path to surgery was long and convoluted. A respondent who found the decision to have surgery very difficult was Irene. 'We discussed the history, the disease, and they said, "We think it's time now for the operation." At that point I was not convinced that I was ready for it, but they said I was, and I remember being very upset, but not tearful that day, and I remember staying calm. I asked them to let me sit and think about it. So they gave me some time. The one thing I did want to know is how serious was it, and that was when they said, "We think that if you leave it any longer it's life threatening." And from that point I said, "Well that's it, that's the decision made, if it's going to be life threatening I have to accept your advice." '

Irene presented her decision as a logical and rational, if very regrettable, outcome of a series of worsening events. By implication, to have behaved differently would have been irrational or illogical. Another respondent who argued in this vein was Shena: 'I couldn't go on any longer. I knew then. The surgeon said it was badly diseased and he said I could have the operation now or in six months. I just stayed. I wasn't leaving. I wanted it done there and then. I didn't think about death but I did think another six months would actually make it worse.' Shena's decision is couched in terms of severity of symptoms, her acceptance of herself as a sick person, and a belief that surgery offered hope. For Shena the disease was the threat. In the next extract Georgina vacillates between defining the disease as the threat and defining the surgery as the threat. 'They started speaking about surgery and I said, "I didn't think it would have to be as extreme as that, you must have other tablets." And that's when they started saying it could be a very serious illness and it could lead to cancer. So I thought, this is a different thing altogether. That's when I realized the seriousness of it. I was crying, but then I got so weak with the colitis, I thought that anything had to be better than this.'

Some of the subjects saw themselves as having gradually come round to the idea. Donna said, 'I think I'm one of those people that just takes time to decide. It wasn't forced on me. I would have had to have it, but I wasn't told you must. I was fortunate. I was asked to take my time and then decide for myself. But the time had come, because I wasn't getting any better. I was coming round to the fact that I would have to have the op. Gradually it got worse and worse and eventually I was just about crawling up the wall.'

Reluctant acceptance of the inevitability of surgery probably comes closest to capturing the typical response. The operation is a last hope or seen as the only hope. Willingness, certainty and fortitude tend not to be the accompanying reactions; resentment and regret are much more likely. Martha described how she felt once operation was recommended: 'I started to think about the kids. All they'd known really was that their mum was sick. They'd gone through this, all through the years and here they were, eight and seven, and I was really sick. I couldn't really do anything. It was hopeless. I was a semi-invalid.' Mary was another person for whom reluctant acceptance of the inevitable best describes her feelings: 'I had known for a year that I was going to have to have a colectomy at some point. I knew the complications.' And Simon, 'I suppose it's the thing to do in a case like mine, just to get it over and done with, at a younger age, rather than wait and put it off. In my case it was so badly inflamed there was no alternative.'

The experience of surgery

Undergoing an operation, any operation, may make people think about themselves in detailed and searching ways. This seems to be particularly so in the case of total colectomy and ileostomy. Subjects talked about the experience in vivid and frequently emotional ways. Surgery was for them a life event of major significance; even with the passage of time it retained a degree of emotional charge which seemed to haunt them, sometimes years afterwards. It is easy to speculate as to the reason why this might be so. The surgery alters the body. The surgery can be extremely painful and post-operative pain can invade and swamp the person. The operation also raises questions of survival. Without it the patient's life will undoubtedly be in danger. Having surgery also carries a risk. These days operative mortality is very low, especially in elective cases. However, the statistics concerning the risk may mean very little to people worrying about their major operation and whether they will pull through. Anaesthesia may be very worrying too. Loss of consciousness may be deeply disturbing.

The initial thing that seemed to concern the respondents was, therefore, the possibility of harm. In terms of the model of coping discussed in Chapter two the focus is on the process of primary appraisal. These are the thought processes dealing with the evaluation of danger. One clear element of danger from the subject's point of view was the possibility of harm. This element could be divided into two: fear of death and fear of pain.

Joyce was worried about dying in the operating theatre: 'I wasn't frightened of what would happen after the operation. I was frightened of *not surviving* the operation. I wasn't frightened of pain, because I thought that pain lessens and pain passes and anyway they can give you pain killers. I knew that I could survive pain. I didn't know if I would survive the operation.' Rhona was also worried about dying: 'People always laugh when I tell them, but I had this terrible fear about dying on the operating table, and I was convinced that the surgeon wouldn't try and save me. I was convinced he would say "Leave her, don't bother resuscitating her."' Christine also thought she would die: 'I said to my husband, "Come up and see me that first night. Wake me and tell me I'm there." I was only frightened of not being there. It was the fact that I might not wake up that I was frightened of.'

Joyce, Rhona and Christine defined the threat as death. Both Joyce and Christine shared their anxieties about dying with their families. They made plans (made clear where their wills were, and left unambiguous instructions as to what to do if they died) and these plans helped them confront their anxieties. All three of these subjects had had very bad symptoms prior to going into hospital and their fears may partly have been grounded in the extreme debilitation they had already suffered. Their coping involved making preparation and sharing their anxieties.

Pain is one of the media whereby people become acutely aware of their body. Whether this is a nagging toothache, chronic back, discomfort, or pain associated with tissue damage in surgery, the experience is keenly felt. In western culture and in medical settings pain is usually negatively evaluated and unsurprisingly, therefore, pain as an assault on the body, indeed as an assault on self, is feared pre-operatively. Gwen's response is illustrative. 'It was just the thought of this operation. Not the fact that I wouldn't come through it, I always thought that if I went while I was on the table, I wouldn't know anything about it, but it was the pain.'

In contrast, Barbara was not so much concerned about pain as about the invasiveness of surgery. 'I wasn't worried about how I was going to look or the bag or anything. It was just the fact of having an operation, of going under an anaesthetic. That's what worried me the most, and things like the tubes they were going to stick down me, and things like that.' The threats of pain or bodily invasion are not easily assuaged. Neither Gwen nor Barbara received any pre-operative counselling about pain and both were left to cope as best they could.

Most adults, within certain broad limitations and with a few exceptions, have a degree of freedom to please themselves about what they do in the minutiae of their life: when to get up in the morning, what to wear, when to have a cup of coffee, for example, are matters of personal choice. Indeed it is in these small details of our everyday lives that we have most freedom to express our personal sense of selfhood. People who have ulcerative colitis are no different from the population at large in this respect except that their symptoms provide an overlay of factors which constrains their choices. However, even rampant symptoms of ulcerative colitis still allow most sufferers to lead lives where they are independent and self-directed, rather than being dependent on other people and controlled by others.

Surgery, and especially its immediate aftermath, drives a metaphorical coach and horses through this independence. Major surgery, like total colectomy, defines the person as dependent on others, albeit transiently. For some people this feeling of being acted upon rather than being self-driven is extremely disturbing. In the next extract, this idea of loss of control is expressed. The respondent is Willie: 'And they were doing something *to you* or *with you*. I remember going into the theatre and getting the big long socks on to keep warm, the injection in the back, counting to about 5. Waking up and saying to the nurse, "Have I been done?" and she told me, "Laddie, you've been done long ago."'

The experience of loss of self, of being acted on rather than acting came through in many other interviews. Joanna, for example, was only 12 years old when she had her operation. The double dependency of being a child and a surgical patient are described. 'Well everything was happening so fast. One minute I was at home, next minute I was in, tests, tubes and X-rays and everything. I was lying there, and all the different doctors and students would be speaking about me, and I didn't know what was happening. The next minute I'd had my operation, there was nothing I could really do.'

It is not only children, however, who are not involved in what is going on. Janet said, 'I was so low. I vaguely remember someone coming and telling me I would need this operation because I'd gone down so quickly. I remember asking if it was cancer. They said about wearing a bag and I said "Yes". If they'd come and told me I'd have two heads, I'd have said "Yes". And that was it, I was just whipped away.' For Janet the loss of independence and loss of self-control was non-problematic and did not require any particular coping because she felt so ill. The only option open to her was submission, indeed she made the point that to behave in any other way would have been foolish.

Surgical wards are geared up to the high dependency needs of their patients. As such the environmental, organizational and inter-personal arrangements serve to set an agenda in which the patient is the dependent party. Some patients experience this as a threat because certain valued aspects of self are devalued. The surgical ward offers cues as to the way patients should behave. It seems to be the case that people experience far less threat if they submit and assume that dependent status. Shena explains this idea. 'I couldn't have cared less. I had no fear. I put my life in Mr Millar's hands, I knew I would be okay with him. I had a lot of respect for him and I didn't feel worried.' John expressed similar sentiments. 'I wasn't in the least worried about it. I was lying on that trolley and my mind was away in the hills. I'd every confidence in that man.'

In the immediate post-operative period, it is not uncommon for the patients to experience a certain sense of non-reality or blunting of experience. That this should be so is unsurprising. The body has suffered extensive tissue damage. At the same time patients have received pain killers which may dull and distort consciousness. In these circumstances some people talk about feeling separated from what is going on. Lizzie explained: 'The Tuesday morning I just lay there waiting for them to take me away to theatre. The next thing I opened my eyes and it was Friday morning. I didn't even know I was away. I felt great. I felt I could've jumped and leapt right out of bed.' Barbara likewise felt somewhat removed from what was happening. 'It was great because I don't remember a thing. I can't remember much. I had these tubes sticking out of me and drips and everything. I suppose it's like when somebody dies. It doesn't hit you at first.'

This sense of distance from what has happened may give way to feelings of relief and a sense of immense well-being. On the basis of these data it is quite impossible to tell whether this euphoria may be explained with reference to the patient's realization of survival, other deep-seated psychological processes, or simply the morphine-based pain relief; what does seem clear, however, is that this may be something of a false dawn. A delayed emotional reaction was reported by some respondents. Andrew, for example, initially made an excellent recovery and seemed to be doing very well. The nursing staff described him as a model patient. He explained what then happened. 'It took a few days for my body to actually realize what had been done to it. I was just living on borrowed time before my body clicked. Something has really been done here. I was then on a downhill slope.'

61

Delayed reaction was a theme mentioned by Rhona. 'When I woke up, I felt so well. It was marvellous. I mean it was the best feeling I've ever experienced. I felt so well. Then, of course, after the first few days you realize just what you've had done. Then, the first time I looked at my scar, I promptly just keeled over. It was such a shock. I used to occasionally stand in front of the mirror and imagine what it would be like to have a stoma, but I always forgot about the scar. I went through a period when I was really down.'

For some people the immediate post-operative response is a shock which is immediate and sudden. Tracy described her experience like this: 'I was lying in my bed and I thought, "What have they done to me?" I was petrified to look down. I was absolutely horrified. "God, they've cut me in half here." I just couldn't look at myself for a good few days, I just absolutely thought it was horrific. It was worse than I ever imagined.' At some point post-operatively patients have to look at what has been done to them, as Tracy mentions. The assault on the body and the self-images this conjures up were described graphically by Irene: 'So on the Wednesday which was two days after my op day, and I had a look. And I'd seen all the stitches, seen this horrible great big bag and all this stuff oozing into it, I felt awful.' Marjorie said, 'I didn't want to touch it, I wouldn't have anything to do with it.'

The general reaction was of surprise and shock. 'I remember when they took off the plaster, the scar seemed an awful size, and the stoma was quite big and swollen. It did look quite ugly for a start' (Mike). 'I remember waking up in intensive care and being very aware of it, aware of tubes everywhere. Nobody warned me that I'd have a nasogastric tube in, I knew I'd have a catheter, I had a cardiac monitor on, and this great big strapping plastic bag. I remember being horrified by the number of tubes' (Mary). All these people had been through a major operation. Their responses suggest that to a significant degree they had been unprepared for their operations. This is surprising given the large numbers of staff and others with an interest in stoma care with whom most of these patients had been in contact prior to the operation.

Some of the people interviewed described their post-operative experiences in terms very like classic grief. Martha's story illustrates the point. 'The first three days were just nothing. I was dead scared to look, really scared. For three days I daren't look down. Then they took me for my first bath. I was absolutely horrified at the scar, this big thing, that's all I could see. After my bath I got back into my bed and I just started crying, I couldn't stop. All I wanted to do was have a good weep. And they wouldn't let me cry. I think I spent two days crying. But it was a combination of everything. I'd seen the bag for the first time, I'd seen the scar.'

Several points about Martha's story may be noted. First, it contains elements of avoidance, denial, feelings of mutilation and weeping which are identified, by, among others, Parkes (1972) as typical of grief. Second, the onset of her reaction occurs some little time after surgery. It is not immediate. It occurred after the physiological process of recovery had begun. In other people's statements the elements of denial, avoidance and mutilation and the difference between psychological and physiological trajectories of recovery and triggers (sometimes unrelated in any direct sense to having surgery) also appear. Bernadette got to seven days post-operatively when she too was asked to have a bath. She had noticed that a cancer patient had previously used the same bath. She became irrational, refusing to get into the bath until it had been thoroughly cleaned. 'Okay, I was being silly, but I felt all my wound was very open, and I was very open. I was vulnerable. I was just beginning to come to terms. I was beginning to realize that this was something I was stuck with for the rest of my life. After I had cleaned the bath myself I got into it. And I sat there, and I sobbed and I sobbed and I wept and I cried. I think I cried for about the whole afternoon. I mean you're different from everybody else. Some people might have had their breast off. But that is nothing to what I had had.' And Mary: 'I remember just lying there thinking God I feel awful and I got more and more upset and things started getting sore, and I just got myself into a terrible state and started crying.'

These extracts, and many others like them, show the extent to which undergoing this operation can be a most shattering experience. It is almost as if there comes a point post-operatively where coping resources become exhausted. The subjects find themselves in a situation which they define as very threatening indeed, but the extent to which they can do anything to cope with it is very limited. The body has been assailed by all kinds of invasive procedures and the patient is more or less powerless to do anything.

Being a new ileostomist

When the person first comes round from anaesthetic after colectomy he or she is now physically an ileostomist, specifically a *new* ileostomist. This newness is reinforced in the ward because patients are not capable of tending their own stoma (for example, emptying their own appliance or changing it). This along with all other body functions are performed on the patient by others. The patient is in a totally dependent position. Perceptually there is no need for the patient to look at the stoma. It will be covered by bed sheets. Mobility may be so severely limited both by post-surgical paraphernalia (tubes, drips, drains and monitors) and by sheer exhaustion, that staring up to the ceiling or sleeping may indeed be the only thing the patient is capable of doing.

Once surgery is over, barring non-routine complications, the role of doctors in the care of patients is limited to monitoring progress. Nurses, on the other hand, spend an enormous amount of time with the patient in the first week or so. The nurses have to care for the patient during the initial period of high dependency, and at that time provide for all the needs of the patient. This can be a very intense relationship. However, as the patient begins to get better, the nurses will spend less time with their charges and then their attention will turn to other patients with greater needs. This is the time when patients are likely to experience extreme emotional reactions to their surgery. The nurse, and the particular organizational context of surgical nursing, routinely impose two different and potentially conflicting identities on the patient – that of very ill post-surgical case needing intensive nursing, and that of recovering but 'cured' patients soon to be discharged. The fact that these two identities may not be compatible and that the patient's emotions may be extremely volatile, sets the scene for highly charged interaction.

Georgina described her experiences thus: 'That was the most horrible experience I have ever had in my life. It was the pain and sickness, it was like a nightmare really. There were days when I just used to cry. You are so weak and tired, and you've got this bag. I said I wasn't very well, and I hadn't slept and he said they would give me antibiotics, and not to lie around. I couldn't have stood and got out of my bed if I'd tried, I'd have fainted. I thought I was never going to get better.' Georgina's hostility was directed at the apparently unsympathetic doctor. Martha's anger was directed at unhelpful nursing staff. She was particularly annoyed about their failure to tell her husband how she was immediately after her operation. 'Joe [her husband] phoned up well into the evening. Nine o'clock at night and he hadn't had any word. I'd gone down to theatre at ten in the morning. So here was all my family left wondering what on earth's happening. Nine was when the night staff came in, who really didn't know anything. Joe phoned and they said I was as well as could be expected. Joe said he wanted to hear more. "Oh that's Sister's policy I'm afraid, we can't tell you anything over the phone." And he was absolutely furious. It's totally wrong. I don't see why they cannot allow your husband to come up just to see you.'

Mary was also angry at the nurses, but because of their ignorance. She had been boarded out, post-operatively to a gynaecology ward. 'Down in the gynaecology ward they didn't have a clue about ileostomy. They didn't know where they were. Sister didn't know how to handle it post-operatively and basically it was lucky that I'd grasped enough about it myself by that stage to know roughly what to do with it myself, because they didn't.' Another respondent who observed that nursing staff were less than helpful was Veronica, who found it impossible to convince the nurses that her appliance needed to be emptied during the night. 'The drip goes twenty-four hours a day, and some of these night nurses said, "Your bowel doesn't work during the night so just go to sleep." I said, "My bowel doesn't know it's night." '

Ambivalence is marked in some of the attitudes to the nursing staff. 'I don't think the nurses deal with you as a person who has had an operation. They are dealing with the actual cut. That's the bit they're concerned with because they don't know about this end product we have, so they can't help you an awful lot in the hospital. But I've had excellent treatment' (Norah). 'In fact I ended up in a ward where there were two young nurses. They'd only come on duty about half an hour before. That was their first stint. I was their first patient. It really gives you a boost – that's not giving any disrespect to them' (Simon). Rhona described what it is like to be neglected once she had begun to recover. 'It must have been after the fifth post-operative day, I was shoved into a side room. I don't see why people with stomas are always palmed off to side rooms. We're not something unacceptable are we?'

The things to note about these patients' immediate reactions to surgery are as follows. The patients are removed physically from their normal social co-ordinates. Their identities as fathers, daughters, workers, bowls players, and friends are superseded by their patient identities. Their surgery leaves them physically weak and in need, for a short while, of total nursing care. At that time they have an identity as an acutely ill post-operative patient. The expectation of the nurses is that they will not remain acutely ill, nor in need of high dependency nursing for very long, and that they will recover. They have been 'cured' of a serious illness and the immediate threat to their lives has been removed. They have a new stoma to deal with. Their emotions may be extreme and their feelings may be complicated by toxic effects, pain and psychological disorientation. The expectations associated with the different identities may be in conflict. In particular the demand of submitting to the role of very sick person in need of high dependency nursing runs counter to the expectations of achieving independence in recovery. The expectations attached to recovery from a serious illness run counter to the expectations linked to living with a permanent incapacity (incontinence). The demands of submitting to the authority of the ward may run counter to many people's habitual independence as adults.

The essence of the new ileostomist's experience in the hospital is identity overlap. The hospital ward demands of them a range of different situated identities. Of course all situations tend to create multiple demands on social actors and a surgical ward is no different from anywhere else in this respect. However, in the surgical ward the options open to the patient are strictly limited. The power of the patient to exert an influence on identity construction and negotiation is highly constrained. In the long run, the patient has the task of coping and of managing his or her stoma. However, what this study has suggested is that the process of acquiring the necessary skills to do this can only be learned once the person is an ex-patient and is at home. For the most part, while the patient is in hospital nursing staff have the responsibility for the care of the stoma.

Even though the patients do not necessarily have to cope with the stoma in a direct sense, they still have to deal with it and other things cognitively, including the contradictory role demands which may be placed on them. At first, when very ill and very dependent, the simplest and most rational course of action is to act sick. However, as new demands are made on the recovering patients they have to take on limited role responsibilities and leave the psychologically comfortable world of the sick role, and emotional conflict may ensue. While their recovery may have begun in earnest, it is often far from clear to them what precisely the expectations of recovery are. Since, at least in the hospitals where these respondents were patients, the routine was for them to be moved to a private side room, all the environmental clues which might help them work out what was required were removed at a stroke. The as yet non-ambulant patients have to second-guess what is required of them from the restricted viewpoint of the side room, a process which many find very difficult. The real business of learning to live with an ileostomy takes place once the patient leaves hospital and the identity of dependent patient is left behind. The nursing staff come in for a lot of flak from the patients, but given the problems the patients are having to cope with, that is hardly surprising.

Parenthetically, it might be added that if dependency continues to be encouraged once the patient gets home, and the individual does not resume other role responsibilities relatively quickly (like going back to work or getting involved with being a father or a mother) the prognosis for a good long term adjustment would probably be poor. The cycle of contradictory identities established in the hospital would be perpetuated.

Sources of help

In an ideal world, in the normal course of events, when a prospective patient is put on the waiting list for surgery a range of para-medical assistance is made available. There are counsellors from the Ileostomy Association, stoma care nurses, stoma therapists and surgical nursing staff, all of whom, along with the surgeon, may have a contribution to make to patient care. As already noted, however, many of the people in this study seemed unprepared, certainly for the magnitude of what happened to them. Commonsensically two reasons suggest themselves for this state of affairs. First, through some organizational problem, prospective surgical cases never got to see appropriate helpers. Second, where help was provided it was either not very good or was inappropriate.

While there might be grains of truth in both these ideas, the explanation is probably more subtle. Recall that many people who had been placed on the waiting list for surgery were themselves extremely reluctant to accept that fact. They vacillated, they resisted and they tried to find excuses for not having the operation. This made them a not particularly receptive group for counselling about post-operative life, because they were resistant to the very idea that there would be a post-operative state at all. Even where people do have accurate information, some find it extremely difficult to anticipate what life is going to be like. 'You think you won't be able to do anything or go anywhere, you imagine all sorts of things, like odour, and that it will be noticeable' (Gwen). Rhona was very worried about a life in which she might be 'well' again. 'I was semi-institutionalized. You were not living a real life. I didn't have any responsibilities. I kept thinking, am I going to be able to manage on my own, how am I going to be able to face up to real life?'

Many patients wanted information and they felt that in spite of the counsellors, visitors and specialists basic information was extremely hard to come by. Gwen said, 'I asked my doctor if he knew anything about it. He said, "All I know is I've met people who've had the operation and they say they feel so much better. I'll try and put you in touch with someone who has had an operation." But it ended up he never did.' Shena tried to find out the difference between an ileostomy and a colostomy but failed to get an answer from her doctor. Marjorie wanted to know whether she would be able to swim but could not find out from her GP.

Bernadette went through the standard nursing preparation in the ward, which she found far from helpful. 'The first thing they did was mark the stoma point and strap a bag to you. And it's quite frightening because you get one of those post-operative bags. They are colossal. It was quite mind boggling really. You are left trying to be blasé and you are left with this bag strapped to you. They didn't tell me what post-operative bags would be like, because they didn't know.'

These data show that the information patients received did not help them work out what having an ileostomy would be like. Their anticipation occurred largely in a situation of information deficit. They could make certain preparations, but these took place in an atmosphere of ignorance. Given that one of the obvious ways of coping with things, especially threatening things, is to collect information, the absence of information, or an inability to make sense of what information is to hand, constitutes a major problem. Small wonder that patients affect resistance up to the last minute; small wonder that their decision-making can be so tortuous; and small wonder that having passed the point of no return that the emotional reaction to the surgery is so intense.

Conclusion

When surgery becomes an immediate prospect the issue for the patient is whether the disease or the operation is the threat. Prospective patients use the full range of coping behaviours from blocking and denial, through information gathering, to bargaining and negotiation to deal with those threats. For some patients who agree to have the operation this involves a rational calculation wherein the benefits of a disease-free future are contrasted with a relatively poor present state of health. For other respondents acceptance of the offer of surgery is really a general reappraisal or sets of reappraisals of events. The principal guiding idea from the point of view of the patient is of the inevitability of the need for surgery. At the heart of the issue for prospective ileostomists are their symptoms. People who believe themselves to be well may be very reluctant to admit that they need surgery. As we saw in the previous chapters, many colitics deny their illness in various ways and in ways which require a major change of their world-view if they are to see themselves as ill. Where symptoms are extremely disruptive of life the reluctant acceptance of the inevitable may be the most logical thing to do.

The prospective surgical patient faces many uncertainties. Information to resolve those uncertainties may for various reasons be unavailable or resisted. Thus the information upon which to base the appraisal, to do the coping, is uncertain too. As the data show, doubts can plague the patient right up to the last minute. When the patient does come to terms with the inevitability of surgery, the uncertainty can be ended. While it may be difficult and even psychologically painful to get to this point, there may well be intense relief that something is at last being done. The patient can then begin the process of re-orienting his or her life to the accomplished fact of the prospective operation.

It is plausible to think of two distinct processes operating independently of each other: election to have surgery and the decision not to have an operation. These two things are not necessarily the opposite of each other, a pair of mutually exclusive alternatives, one of which is positive and one negative. Both are actually positive decisions. Both groups – those who elect and those who refuse – have positive reasons for doing what they do. The question of election or refusal is not about the absence or presence of particular information nor about its distortion, it is about the individuals changing their view of themselves so that they define themselves as sick. The process involves giving up old strategies for living and coping with the disease and an acknowledgement of the inevitability of the operation because the alternatives to having surgery are regarded as worse than surgery or worse than the ileostomy. The process is one of aligning the self with the public identity of prospective and actual surgical case.

In the psychological literature on surgery the way coping skills relate to surgical outcome has received much attention. Cohen and Lazarus (1973) compared patients who avoided or denied the threatening aspects of surgery with patients who were vigilant, that is, who deliberately sought out information. They suggested that patients showing a vigilant mode of coping generally showed a slower rate of recovery, while avoiders did best. This argument was placed against the then conventional wisdom about surgical recovery from a psychological point of view which was associated with the work of Janis (1958). Janis had suggested that patients with moderate levels of fear would be less likely to develop post-surgical emotional problems. Andrew (1970) produced data supportive of the idea that recovery from surgery can be influenced by psychological preparation. Elsewhere Janis argued that there is a relationship between intensity of fear arousal and adaptive coping responses (Janis, 1974; Langer et al., 1975; Langer, 1983: 137; Janis, 1985).

Much has been written about pain and its relationship to surgery. In a much quoted paper Egbert and associates reported that they were able to reduce the amount of reported pain and requests for pain relief by using placebo methods, by instruction and by showing an interest in surgical patients (Egbert et al., 1964: 825–7). What does not seem in doubt is that patients in this study reported acute pain in their responses; it is equally clear that their pre-operative counselling had not prepared them for this. However, whether more elaborate pre-operative counselling would have made any difference is quite impossible to gauge from this study.

There is a hefty literature on counselling. In general it has been argued that counselling should aim to help by telling people what to expect from forthcoming traumatic events (Moos and Tsu, 1977: 18). Hazards, so the argument goes, may be attenuated because they have been made familiar by being anticipated (Caplan, 1964: 84). Many of the patient education booklets for prospective colectomy patients pay lip service to this approach although given the information deficits reported by these respondents, the model of 'attenuating the threat' does not necessarily work very well in practice.

Of the responses provided by the patients the most striking thing is the emotional intensity of the experience which is reported. Although not developed specifically in respect of surgery of the gut, nor indeed of surgery of any description, the loss and grief processes described by writers such as Parkes (1972) have a resonance with the hospital experiences described by some of the patients. It was Lindemann whose early work provided the bench-mark. On the basis of the clinical observations of the bereaved and of disaster victims, he argued that acute grief is a definite syndrome with both psychological and somatic symptoms, including tightness in the throat, choking, shortness of breath, sighing, empty feelings in the abdomen, loss of muscular power and mental distress (Lindemann, 1944). Lindemann introduced the concept of grief work which means breaking the bond to the lost person and readjusting to and coping with the new environment. This involves working through the grief in order for something like a normal life to resume.

The important work of Parkes (1972) suggests that grief resembles a physical injury more than any other type of illness. It is, he argues, a functional psychiatric disorder with a distinctive and predictable course, through numbness, pining and depression, to recovery. Parkes suggests that grief is rooted in separation and the breaking of a strong bond of attachment. Alarm is one aspect of the response and is characterized by definite physical changes in the central nervous system and high levels of arousal. Searching is another phase, associated with episodic and acute pangs of grief and pining. Numbness, feelings of unreality and blunting are frequently juxtaposed with searching behaviour and these constitute attempts to mitigate or to avoid the pain of grief. It is a way of acting as if the loss had not happened and may allow valuable time to prepare for the full meaning of the loss to be realized. Anger and guilt are important components of grief, although these emotions change with the passage of time. Coming to terms with loss involves *coping* by finding new meanings in life. The similarities between the grief processes and those described by the respondents, coupled with the fact that some who had been bereaved readily acknowledge the similarity of bereavement to the feeling of loss after surgery, highlight an interesting connection between the two experiences.

While the process of emotional healing may be described in terms of the dynamics of loss and bereavement, it should also be noted that this process is not apparently related in a direct causal way with the process of physical recovery. In a very crude sense what seems to happen is that in the very immediate post-operative period, say the first four or five days, while the body's own physiological recovery processes become operative, patients can enjoy a certain amount of psychological equanimity. The emotional surge seems to occur around about a week post-operatively. By this time, not infrequently the physical healing processes are well under way, then and only then can or does the emotional healing seem to begin.

Not all patients reported the grief-like reactions. One might speculate that the reason for this lies in the fact that given the highly personal and indeed personally threatening nature of admitting to weeping and crying, some subjects were simply unwilling to disclose what they really went through. However, perhaps some people simply do not experience the grief-like feelings. Whether in the long run they would be any better or worse adjusted to their surgery could only be demonstrated by a very different kind of study from this one. However, anecdotally, and coincidentally there seems some validity in the view that those patients who 'worked through' their feelings in something akin to a grief reaction seemed to be rather better adjusted, or at least to be more at peace with themselves, than those who argued, sometimes vehemently, that they were fine and always had been fine.

In terms of the overall model of coping which will be developed in the final chapter of this book, two elements from the experience of surgery are important. First, coping both with the prospect of surgery and with surgery itself involves a change in self – people undergoing that change have to bring their personal sense of who and what they are into line with the public identity bestowed on them by virtue of their diagnosis and the medical opinion that they need surgery. Second, this experience is a profoundly disturbing one, a major life event which mimics the loss–grief paradigm described particularly by psychoanalytically oriented writers in respect of bereavement. The transition in self involves processes of 'working through' to resolution. Coping, in other words, involves intense emotional work and, while surgery is quintessentially a physical event, in certain cases, of which colectomy is one, the emotional charge attached thereto is considerable.

Chapter five

Living with an ileostomy

After the initial surgical trauma and the ups and downs of the early post-operative months the now ex-patient has to settle down to something approaching an ordinary life. He or she can go back to work, can take up favoured leisure activities, and can resume a normal diet. The person has been cured of a major illness and although the experience of surgery may have been quite devastating, can look forward to a new disease-free existence. Yet the ex-patient still has to cope with the ileostomy. In this chapter the problems of a life with an ileostomy are documented.

People who have newly acquired an ileostomy are the same people as they were when they had colitis. They are the same age, gender, occupation and marital status, with the same address, the same dispositions, sense of humour and educational qualifications, for example. By all the standard identity markers they are the same people that they were pre-operatively. The exception to this is that they are cured of their disease. They are not, however, returned to their pre-morbid situation; they are cured, but they are different. Moreover, ileostomist is a definite social as well as medical category. It carries with it certain (if ill-defined) social expectations. It entails membership of a particular category of persons who are distinguished from others by their possession of a stoma. That stoma has a freight of more or less socially significant connotations. It is not, however, publicly visible. Other people cannot see it, unless the ileostomist is undressed. Theoretically, when functioning properly the ileostomy should not be a major handicap. There is no physical disability in terms of loss of function or mobility, and therefore the impact on post-operative life is potentially minimal.

Living with the new stoma

The first thing which must be learned is how to wear, use, and change an appliance. These skills are often acquired with some difficulty. Help is usually available from nurses and others, including more experienced people with ileostomies. However, the basic micro finger skills are quite complicated. Also they have to be learned when most people are not at their most receptive nor their most able. They are in a hospital ward, they feel ill or depressed, or they have just got home and feel weak and tired. The ex-patient is a novice who has to learn everything from scratch.

Tracy described the problems like this: 'Then in addition you've got the practical aspect of looking after it. You've got to learn a new language. It's materials you've never seen in your life, equipment you've never known existed, names you've never heard of, a routine that seems so alien, it's so strange.' Pauline explained: 'I remember the first time I had a bath in hospital, they decided that they were going to change it. The bags you get in hospital, they've got the brown stuff round and it all sticks to you, and it wouldn't come off, and it was all over the bath water, I started crying in the bathroom, it was horrible.' John emphasized the difficulties: 'You start thinking about how you are going to cope. You are told about the different fittings, you have to cope with it and you've got to learn very quickly.'

Some patients seem to get a great deal of help when learning how to use their new appliance. Christine is a case in point: 'Sister saw that I knew what I was doing, and how! before I left there. And I had my clothes on in the ward before I went home to see how I would do. She made sure I was right!' Benny was also very pleased with the help he got. The first time it was changed he was concerned, ' "God, do I have to go through this every time?" That was when the nurses were doing it. Then the stoma therapist came up, which was a revelation: little white bag, lot smaller, lot neater, lot more compact, went into a little cotton bag. I asked her to show me what to do. And that was it.'

While Benny and Christine were happy with the coaching they received, several other respondents were not. 'No, there was no help I got. While I was in the ward you just got told "Right, use it, you learn to use it yourself, for you've got to use it yourself when you go home, do it, get on with it." Nobody came to see me' (Stella). This lady had had her surgery more than twenty years before she was interviewed, and indeed in those days support services were not very highly developed. Annie was operated on only months before she was interviewed. She fared little better, however. 'You were just bunged out of hospital, that was it, you were told just to carry on with it, make the best of things. I was told in the hospital, it was only in about a day or two after the operation, "Change that yourself. Have you ever done it?" And I said, "no". "Oh well you'll need to start doing it now." That was it.'

Sally likewise received hardly any help at all, to the extent that the original appliance she received in the operating theatre was left in place for several weeks. The potential for skin damage would have been considerable. 'Well the bag had never been changed. I had never looked at it, and they did not seem perturbed about it either. Now that was about three weeks and that bag had never been touched, never been changed.' Some of the respondents reacted quite positively to being left alone to get on with it. Barbara, for example, said, 'From the second day I was doing everything myself, well I was wanting to and they just let me. I don't know myself how I coped, but I just did!'

Learning to change and use an appliance was perceived by most respondents to have been tricky at first, but something which, with perseverance, could be mastered quite quickly. What these extracts show is that while all subjects did indeed learn to manage to cope with their bags, the extent to which they perceived others as providing help was very varied. Where help was not forthcoming, and it was wanted, this was very much resented.

When patients first leave hospital and they go home they usually have to change their appliance themselves. They are still learning about the intricacies of appliances, how they fit together and which appliance system is most suitable for them. In these circumstances changing an appliance can appear to be a daunting task. Patients at that time are quite weak and can tire easily. Standing in the bathroom for about half an hour to change can be exhausting (it takes someone with experience considerably less time to change an appliance, but not so the novice).

The next problem novices have to deal with is the permanence of the presence of their appliance and its unpredictable potential for leaking. People who have ileostomies always need to have access to replacement appliances in case the one they are wearing fails. Most carry spare appliances with them or secrete them around the place (in the car, in desk drawers and such like) so that they can execute a quick change in case of an emergency. If they go on holiday, on a trip, or go to stay at a hotel or someone's house, they will need to take spares with them. If they find themselves in a situation where they have no spare appliances, and they have a leak or the bag falls off, they would have to stay in reach of a receptacle to catch their faeces, which will run in a more or less continuous stream. Without an appliance the person cannot function. In the early post-operative days, appliance failure tends to be very common. This is partly because of the inexperience in putting them on properly, and partly because some novices do not recognize the warning signs of an impending leak and fail to react in time.

For Bert the problem was getting an appliance to stick on at all. 'You had to take the back off, stick it down, take the bottom half off and then take the two little bits off the side and then stick that down. I'm afraid I used to have a few cursings and swearings in the bathroom because sometimes it didn't stick properly and I had to take it off again, and go away and get a new one.' Tracy said, 'The only thing that I find slightly difficult is putting the karaya seal on, which is pretty sticky and then all the time I have a bit of gauze over the stoma, and then trying to get a bag and just quickly put it over it before it runs down my leg.'

The fact that unpredictable leaks can be controlled if caught in time was emphasized by Marjorie. 'Oh I'm aware when something's gonna happen. It's my fault if something happens, it's 99 per cent my fault.' The more routine aspects of changing appliances are illustrated by Gwen. 'I've no bother with keeping bags on. I find it quite easy. With my appliance there is a face and a wafer thing to start with and then the bag itself. With the other one I used, you needed a wafer, a karaya ring and then a bag, and then you had to put the clip on the bag and it didn't take long. I usually change it every three days, but I could actually go longer than that, I could. I could go four or five. The thing I find awkward is disposing of the bags when you are away from home, y'know it's a bit awkward, you don't like to dump them in somebody's bin.'

Skill in changing the appliance is basic to having an ileostomy. Without this skill, someone with an ill-fitted appliances can be seriously restricted in mobility and hence other activities. A properly fitted appliance and the knowledge that the person with an ileostomy has of any problem the appliance might present, allow it eventually to become a background feature of life.

Normal but different

Someone with an ileostomy defecates differently from other people. His or her stoma has no voluntary muscular involvement so is active without the individual having control over it. This activity happens at any time: when walking, talking, eating, sleeping, travelling, and going to church. In any occupation in which the person is engaged he or she may be defecating at the same time. Uncontrolled defecation would, in the normal course of events, be regarded as a transgression of social convention. However, the individual who has an ileostomy is in the strange situation of being different in this respect, but of that difference usually being unknown and unobservable to others. Occasionally a stoma may make a noise caused by flatulence, but it does not sound like a person breaking wind, so does not offend that particular convention.

At the same time as the ileostomy is producing faeces it is being collected in the appliance. Much of the time people with an ileostomy will be walking around with a quantity of faeces on their person. This too is a secret unobservable to others. These differences have to be incorporated into these people's long-term notion of who and what they are (their self). These differences are not transient and unimportant; they are permanent and they are symbolically significant. The way some individuals handle this is to emphasize the normal ordinary aspects of themselves as people, rather than focusing on the ileostomy. Harry said, 'I play hockey once a week and I don't find it exhausting or tiring, I play squash, badminton, and tennis. I don't find I'm restricted because of my bag.' Maggie also emphasized sporting activity. 'This lady who I used to play with was unaware I had an ileostomy and she said, "I play badminton with you every week" and I mean I wore my little white skirt and everything, she said, "You run about and you jump"; it didn't get me down at all.'

This is not to say that acting normally and emphasizing activities which aim to stress ordinariness, are easy. Doubts and uncertainties may be important parts of the learning process. 'The first couple of days I was home I wondered whether I was going to be able to get back into the swing of it, to wear nice clothes and dress up, go out and do the shopping. But it all happened. It all came about in no time, and it's great, it's great to be able to do it all again' (Joyce).

However, acting normally and engaging in activities which stress good health, are both contingent on the stoma and the appliance functioning properly. It was noted above that appliance failures tended to be more common for the novice than for the experienced user. There are other problems which are commonly encountered which emphasize the distinctiveness of someone with an ileostomy both to themselves, and to others. Diet is one of the principal problem areas.

Physiologically there is no reason why having an ileostomy should be a barrier to eating a normal diet, with the proviso that someone with a stoma may be deficient in water and sodium and therefore should drink slightly more fluids than non-ileostomists and take additional salt in the diet. However, in spite of the physiology some foods sometimes cause blockages. What happens is that a bolus of partially digested food plugs the stoma or the ileum. Debilitation can be rapid and hospital admission may be required. This possibility means that diet may be an issue of continuing concern. Peter explained. 'If you eat certain foods, like peanuts, and you don't digest them properly and it builds up in the bowel it forms a blockage – skins, or cabbage that hasn't been cooked properly. You get excruciating pains. In fact I had to ask the doctor in once.' Julie alluded to a similar type of problem: 'It depends what I eat really. I use trial and error. Sprouts have to be well cooked, but if I eat five or six of them I'm apt to leak because it goes into a mass and just goes out underneath the appliance. I ate macaroons once, and all they consist of is just coconut; it was four I ate; by the middle of the night I had really colicky pain. I realized what had happened so I kept drinking fluids. I was in a lot of pain. The doctor came and eventually I went to hospital. I don't think they quite knew what to do. Someone came down and I explained. They took a glass tube and even that wouldn't dislodge it.' Janet took precautions in what she ate. 'I always peel my tomatoes. And oranges I've found aren't that great. I've never even attempted an apple with the skin on.' And finally Ron: 'I used to steer clear of oranges and onions, and once with a very hot curry I was really ill. But these last few years I don't think there is anything I can't take. I've never tried oranges, grapefruit yes, but oranges no. I've tackled everything else including whisky, gin, brandy, sherry, beer, anything.'

Diet and the possible consequences of dietary indiscretion serve as a constant reminder of the ileostomy. Direct experience of a blockage and the accompanying acute pain, diarrhoea and dehydration serve as signal reminders of distinctiveness. This becomes a constant part of the background to life. Sometimes there maybe a trade-off between risking a favourite food, like peanuts or curry, and the possible negative outcome. The first time a blockage occurs it may be very alarming. However, because most blockages are self-limiting, many people cope with their diet by continuing to take occasional dietary risks, calculating that in the long run little harm will come to them. From a social-psychological point of view dietary attention is a constant background feature of self, the background reminder of the thing that makes them different or distinct.

The stoma and the appliance are objects of attention and annoyance but in general they can become background features of everyday existence. However, from time to time they can become extremely intrusive. When dietary problems occur or when buying clothes, when having a bath or shower, the appliance is noticeable. The stoma and appliance demand attention when they need to be cleaned and changed. The ileostomy is obvious every time the individual goes to the toilet.

However, these things in themselves could scarcely be judged to be tragic life events, and neither should they be activities which produce high levels of anxiety. At least according to these respondents, they need not be. So long as everything is working, it is low-grade awkwardness, intrusiveness and obviousness and minor adjustments to life that are the lot of someone with an ileostomy. Coping skills are certainly required, but once learned (for example, how to change an appliance, what sort of clothes can be worn in comfort, what foods to avoid) the threat posed to routine functioning by the ileostomy is minimal. The coping process is one in which the ileostomy can be customarily appraised as something benign or irrelevant. Unsurprisingly, subjects who had had their ileostomy a long time were the ones most likely to see it as benign or irrelevant. 'Living with this ileostomy with these modern bags is just nothing. No one knows I have it. As far as I'm concerned I don't have it. I don't know I've got it' (Joyce, who was very experienced). However, even those who have had their appliances for less than a year may adopt a similar attitude. 'You forget about it, and you are not aware of anyone with it. For most of the time I don't even think about it' (John, who had had his operation within the previous year). 'I'm amazed how I've adapted to it, I forget that I've got it at times. It's not until I feel the bag getting heavy or swollen that I realize there's something there' (Susan, who had had her operation about six months before interview).

Accidents

Unfortunately accidents can and do occur. Appliances become detached and fall off. Many leak periodically. The possibility of appliances becoming completely unstuck, and the more common problem of leakage, are things that must be prepared for. Willie explains: 'I've had the occasional flurry of things not quite going right, like the bag dropping off. That used to bother me, but it doesn't now. If that happens it doesn't bother me.' Gwen describes the experience of leaks. The following incident occurred at night; this is very common. It occurs because the person is lying horizontally and the contents of the bag are likely to leak under the part of the appliance which is attached to the skin. It is less likely to happen when the person is walking about and standing upright because the contents settle at the bottom of the bag away from the skin and are hence less likely to ooze out. Gwen said, 'It happened the first time I went away after my operation. I woke up at three o'clock in the morning and the bag had started to leak. It happened two nights later'. Fred said, 'There was a leak the other night. It was my own fault. It needed to be emptied and I just couldn't be bothered to get up. I leaned over and it came off.' Caroline confided, 'Three times it's burst or come off in bed. Where do you start to clean up? The smell is terrible. That's why I don't go to bed early. I'm frightened to.'

In order to cope, the person with an ileostomy has to estimate the danger of a leak or of an accident. It is more likely to occur if the bag needs to be changed and if the adhesive seal is becoming less effective. It is more likely to happen at night if the bag is full and if the motion is very liquid. Each of these risks can be controlled by direct actions like changing the appliance, emptying the appliance before going to bed and avoiding those foods which cause a liquid motion. The issue is more difficult if someone is away from home when a leak occurs. Even here, putting a bath towel in the bed to sleep on would avoid most of the mess from a leak. These routine preventive actions, which are the means of dealing with the threat posed by potential leaks and accidents, must become part of the texture of self. This is not to say they become a constant preoccupation, although for some people they may do. Rather, it is to argue that in order to cope, people with an ileostomy cannot simply breeze along without thinking about the consequences of their stoma and the way it might impinge on the other things they may want to do.

The routines though are simple and pragmatic, as the next quotations illustrate. 'I just watch what I eat. I avoid the things that don't agree with me' (Norman). 'When I'm working I always have spares with me, and I carry a bag with me as an emergency supply' (Fred). 'The first time you are away from home you are always frightened of a leak in the night. You can put a towel down to make sure, but you can't always sleep properly because you get a bit tense' (Julie).

Accidents need to be coped with. They demand either anticipating actions to obviate threat in the case of potential accidents, and they demand readily available towels, spare clothes, and replacement appliances when accidents do occur. In terms of their feelings about themselves taking such precautions is not so much seen as normal, that is, what other people do, but rather the sort of thing anyone would do in order to maintain a sense of normality. And it is that sense of trying to present a normal external appearance to others in order to construct a normal identity, which for the self involves a recognition of the break from normality.

Visibility

Someone who has an ileostomy looks normal when fully dressed, but they are different underneath; they know this even if the majority of others are unaware of the stoma. Keeping the appliance out of sight is important to maintain the veneer of normality. Mostly, the true nature of the ileostomy and its appliance are irrelevant for normal social functioning. Substantial and permanent identities like age, gender, occupation and most identities relating to situations like being a customer, a passenger, a pedestrian or a football match spectator can all be accomplished without any reference to the ileostomy. This is true as long as the appliance is not visible.

In the early days after coming out of hospital respondents indicated that they could hardly believe that other people could not see the appliance. 'I found I was worried about meeting people for the first time. I thought it was a very obvious thing. I felt I couldn't walk along the street but everyone would see this huge bump and realize I had a bag. But of course you soon realize not a soul even turns a hair' (Jean). 'The first day I went out I lost all my confidence. I was convinced that when I walked down the high street people would look at me and say, "Look at her, what a shame she's got a bag." I couldn't believe that people wouldn't be able to see it' (Marjorie).

These two extracts show that soon after surgery the presence of the stoma can cause a good deal of anxiety, but that quickly the realization occurs that when one is dressed, the appliance is easily concealed. There are certain leisure activities, especially those involving going into public changing facilities, which can cause concern. The responses to this vary from openly brazening it out: 'I half hoped somebody would turn round in the shower and say "What's that you've got on your side?" and I'd be ready to retort, "Well would you come into a shower if you had this?" ' (Harry), to withdrawal from situations where such complications or their potential would not occur: 'After squash I just say I'll go back home and have a shower in the house' (Tom). Keeping the appliance out of sight and, therefore, of no salience or relevance in interaction is a routine accomplishment basic to having an ileostomy and one which helps to maintain a normal identity.

Complications

Surgical and long-term medical complications constitute problems for some. 'My stoma has sunk in a hole. I can have it resited, which is the last alternative because they have only one more place to put it, that's on top of my scar, so the chances are that my guts will fall out. So I can either put up with several leaks a day or have another operation' (Rhona). However, major problems of this type were not common among the respondents in this study. Minor surgical complications were, though, particularly slow healing of the perineal wound. 'I've always had this problem with the back passage wound which has been leaking since I had the operation. I've been in at least three or four times since and it's never really healed. Its horrible. It leaves a smell which isn't very nice' (Jane).

One important point about stomal and perineal complications is that in their way they can be as intrusive and as unpredictable as the symptoms of ulcerative colitis. They can spoil identity construction. This occurs both in the sense that public performance may be discredited and also they prevent the resumption or continuation of normal activities post-operatively. When complications occur they have to be coped with.

Diarrhoeal dehydration (of infectious origin) is another complication. Caroline described it thus: 'The bag was just filling up and filling up, and it was just like lime juice. I got light headed and sick and I kept passing out. I got cramp in my legs. I had to go to hospital and get on the drip.' Straightforward dehydration brought on by heat is another possible problem. 'I have to watch and not get dehydrated in warm weather. Once or twice if I've been on holiday and I haven't had a place where I could get a drink of water and I've started to feel woozy' (Janet).

When these things happen they correspond to a classical acute episode of symptom–intervention–relief–recovery. Most such episodes are self-limiting. However, although they tend to be transient they may be common occurrences. Self-medication of electrolyte imbalance restoring fluids is an obvious intervention and having such things available is a wise precaution. The fact that self-medication may be ineffective and rapid dehydration can be very serious, leads a few people to carry a tag around their necks like diabetics, to indicate their potential problem. Some members of the Ileostomy Association recommend taking a partner along to all consultations where dehydration is the problem, just in case the ileostomist loses consciousness altogether and an inexperienced doctor fails to recognize the problem.

The other common medical complication is skin deterioration. Skin deterioration around the stoma is caused by the digestive enzymes in the excrement attacking the skin, or the skin reacting to the appliance or to the tapes or adhesives holding the appliance in place. Martha's experience is illustrative. 'First there was a bit of skin starting to break down, but I didn't run to the doctor. Of course it gradually got worse. It got that bad that the appliance wouldn't stick. I had to have time off work again, and I was off another six months. The skin would not clear up. I felt as if my whole world was just crashing about me.' Janet also had severe problems, 'Oh boy, did I have a sore skin. At one stage, I was cutting the plastic, I was cutting a section away at a time to try to let that bit heal before I went on to the next bit because it was so bad. The bags wouldn't stick for any length of time.'

Successful management of life with an ileostomy involves taking precautions to ensure appliances do not leak. However, even the most careful precautions cannot always prevent skin reactions. If such reactions can be treated or self-treated promptly then there is no real difficulty. If the problem is not treated and it worsens, after a while it becomes impossible for an appliance to stick on at all. This means the individual is virtually disabled, perhaps housebound, and certainly many activities will need to be curtailed. Simply keeping an appliance on becomes a major task. Thus problems of self-image, identity presentation, embarrassment and the awareness of others of the appliance immediately become foreground issues. Some people with stomas tread a fine line between functional limitation and normality, because their skin is a chronic problem. Medically speaking the skin breakdown is a minor lesion, but its social implications can be major.

Relationships

The person with a stoma is part of a network of family, friends, working relationships and leisure activities. There is no reason why someone with an ileostomy should not earn a living nor engage in ordinary leisure activities. Many ex-patients pick up these aspects of their lives post-operatively and work and play like anybody else. Some jobs might be excluded, for example, being a nude model might present problems and doing a job that involved a lot of very heavy lifting might be ill-advised. A few leisure activities, especially contact sports like rugby or boxing, are dangerous not only intrinsically but also because of the likelihood of physical damage to the stoma. Some ileostomists seem to do them anyway. However, the ileostomy is of little or no relevance in most jobs or most leisure activities.

Relationships, especially sexual relationships, are areas of considerable concern. These worries tend to be voiced pre-operatively; they also tend to surface post-operatively. In the interviews a range of responses to the question of sexual relationships arose. First Jean, who claimed her ileostomy was irrelevant: 'The boyfriends have accepted it as well, and have not seen it as a problem, because I have not seen it as a problem, so in my personal relationships it's no problem.' Tracy was outgoing and direct and seemed to take the view that her boyfriend had to take her as she was; the men who did not like her stoma, she claimed, would not be worth knowing anyway. Mary saw things rather differently. 'How could I be going out with someone and say, "I've got something to tell you". I have a fear of somebody turning round and saying "Oh yeah" and going out the door and never coming back.' Mike's philosophy was to be open and frank. 'If you are getting into a sexual situation, you are best to let your partner or prospective partner know what the score is.' John was more circumspect. 'I was still an unmarried man. I was a little bit reluctant to ask a girl out or whatever. I decided that the best thing to do was to go out with the girl several times over the space of a month or something, go out three or four times. If you were beginning to get to the stage where you liked them that was as good a point as any to explain. I'd say I had a slightly unusual body design and I had a bag on my side. I also made a point of showing it to them.'

In the next two extracts Jane and Barbara, neither of whom were married, put the open philosophy into practice, or tried to, and suffered as a consequence. 'When you do meet somebody, and if you like him, well I feel they should know. But it's trying to tell them, I find it very very hard. Where do you start telling them? Where do you begin? I just seem to crack up, and the tears start to come.' 'I told this boy and he said it didn't matter and that his grandad had had the same operation. But the next time he saw me, he never spoke to me. That really put me off. My last boyfriend, I told him, and he sat back and said, "God what's this, I'm really shocked." But he accepted it. I'm not going out with him now. We fell out about something else.'

Undoubtedly respondents who did not have partners voiced considerable anxieties about their ileostomies. Most succinctly, Rhona put it like this: 'I am eighteen years old. Who's gonna love me with this?' However, those who are married also have problems, anxieties and worries. 'I looked at my body, and I saw the big scar and this at the side. And I thought will my husband ever look at me again?' (Susan). But many seem to reach a reasonably satisfactory way of living with the bag. 'As far as sexual life's concerned it's never made one iota of difference between Kate and I. Kate never pushed me one way or another. And now it's just as normal as you can be with a bag. You've got to empty it before sex, but it's never affected us that way' (Bert).

What is clear from the transcripts is that the way sexuality is handled by doctors and nurses was regarded, by these respondents, as not very helpful. Rhona argued, 'The doctors kept saying that I'd be able to have a normal sex life, and have a family. That made me angry because I'm not an appendage of a man or child.' Marjorie said, 'They seemed to be very concerned about my sex life and kept telling me I could have a normal sex life. But there was no boyfriend, so why bother?'

Sexual relationships are an important component of people's identities and their sense of self. In the youthful age group, where colitis and ileostomy are most likely to occur, these concerns may be heightened. The transcripts show, not surprisingly, that sexual relationships are a source of anxiety, particularly for the unmarried or unpartnered. As people in this situation appraise it, of all the dangers they can identify sexual rejection is one of the most important. Rejection is not just a blow to self-image, it is also a genuine assault on identity. Being sexually active involves significant others legitimizing certain claims made by self. At the heart of people's concern is the fear that the legitimacy of themselves as sexual beings will be denied by rejection. The way people cope in these situations can take a number of forms: by being frank or honest, by trying to find the right moment, or by simply withdrawing.

The above quotations suggest that the notions of rejection are tied in with notions of being sick. Thus, despite what these subjects have been told (that they can have a normal sex life) and in spite of the advice which is more or less universally given (that they should be frank with potential and actual sex partners), identities can be assigned by potential and actual partners which do not take account of these things. The identity which may be assigned by them is that of sick person, non-normal and non-legitimate sex partner. This is ultimately a biological contingency, because whatever efforts the person who has an ileostomy makes at self presentation, his or her own awareness of others' potential identity assignations limits the transformation of identity involved in moving from colitic to ileostomist.

The issues surrounding sexuality are to some extent a microcosm of relationships in general. In relationships with significant others and in general social relations someone with an ileostomy has to consider how much information it is necessary to reveal to other people and under what circumstances. When the ileostomy is functioning normally and when there is otherwise good health, there is no need for the person to reveal anything in routine interaction. When statuses and roles are involved in which the only salient identity is that of adult male or adult female, the presence of the ileostomy is irrelevant, to all intents and purposes. However, in certain other types of situation the person with an ileostomy may be obliged to disclose the truth: in a sexual encounter, a medical examination, a body search at an airport, applying for life insurance and so on.

Between these situations where disclosure is necessary and those where the ileostomy is irrelevant, there are a range of other circumstances where people with an ileostomy have a choice and can exert some degree of control over the flow of information about themselves which may in turn have implications for their identity. The fact of revelation could be distressing because it could result in harm, loss or threat (embarrassment, ridicule, rejection, destruction of relationships or spoiling of preferred identities). In such circumstances the way of coping with this is to act and appear normal, and to conceal the ileostomy. Given that in many, if not most, situations passing oneself off as normal is not likely to be challenged, this is a low-risk strategy.

However, in some cases they may conclude that revelation may carry positive benefits, like eliciting sympathy or praise. If the person with an ileostomy believes that he or she will be able to manipulate others by revelation, then coping may take the form of revealing information. This is a more high-risk activity, because while it *may* attract the desired identity legitimation, it may also attract ridicule, rejection and spoiled identity.

The person with an ileostomy therefore has to make a decision about revelation. There is no rule of thumb which can be applied in every circumstance, and each situation has to be appraised on its merits. What seems to be the case is that the greater the preoccupation the person has about his or her ileostomy, that is, the greater the degree of salience it has for self, the greater seems to be the likelihood that information will be revealed to others about the ileostomy, thus making it an issue of importance in identity construction. The whole process may become more complicated if the person loses control over information flow. Pauline had a particularly unfortunate experience in this regard. 'I went out, and this girl asked me how I was feeling; I said I was fine. I thought seeing that I live in such a small town, I thought she'd heard I'd been in hospital, and I thought that's as far as the conversation would go. But she said, "That's a terrible operation you've had, how do you cope with that bag?" And I hadn't told anyone outside my family. I asked her how she found out. "Oh my sister's a staff nurse in theatre." '

Kathleen in contrast seemed to take the process of revelation to extremes. 'In the village I have been visited, and I say I've got a bag. And I don't feel embarrassed because they are really interested. And to really close friends I've shown the appliances too.' Others are more cautious. 'I don't go out and tell people. I wouldn't go out and say I'd had that done, but I wouldn't be bothered about people knowing, it doesn't bother me' (Janet). 'I can't really face telling anyone about it. People keep saying to me it's nothing to be ashamed of, but I just don't feel ready to tell anyone about it. So no one actually knows apart from my family' (Frances).

Pauline, who found that people in a small town were gossiping about her, is referring to a problem that someone with an ileostomy may face in any community or group, where their absence over a period of time may excite comment. Many work-places, for example, can have the characteristics of small communities, and employing organizations may be privy to the physical status of the ileostomist, because of sickness certification. The transcripts show that there is no consistent pattern of experience. Geoff, for example, found he was shunned by his former workmates: 'When Jim Jones came round just after New Year he asked what was wrong. I told him. He backed off, he virtually ran out the door. I'd hardly got the beer out, the whisky. And I'd known him for years.' Bert found he was transferred to 'lighter', less demanding work. 'I'd been in the police nineteen years. The Chief Superintendent came up one day when I was still off and he said, "We want to make a Crime Prevention Officer out of you." ' Martin went back to work on the railways, but switched from working on goods trains to working on passenger trains, so that he would have access to toilets. 'I just stick to passenger trains so I can easily get to a toilet. There's no problem that way.'

For some respondents getting back to work was a struggle because employers put obstacles in their way. Ron was a master mariner. 'I went to see the doctor before going back to sea. He said, "I'm very sorry but you are certainly permanently unfit to go back to sea." I said, "You'd better think again." They decided to give me a trial on the home trade. I said, "That's no bloody good." So they decided I could go to the tropics. I went to the West Indies. I felt all right. I had no trouble, no bother. And I was at sea for another sixteen years till I had a heart attack.' In Ron's case his problems were from his current employer. In Christine's case the problems were from a prospective employer. She had passed an examination to become a teacher and then had to go for a medical. 'After the medical I was told that they had decided that I wouldn't be able to do it. I was told I wasn't fit. It was really one slap in the face for me.'

These quotations mirror the issues in sexuality. Significant others, in this case employers, are in a position to define identity in particular ways independent of the self-presentational efforts of the subjects. Identity construction is to some extent negotiable but the partners in the identity construction are not equal. For some, this unequal struggle meant that in the long run they gave up working altogether, especially where the employer was unsympathetic. 'I have had to stop work because I wasn't getting my right sleep. And I didn't have the same energy that I used to have. I got tired very quickly' (Caroline).

Accounts

Some of the subjects were very unhappy, angry and resentful about their experiences. 'I lost eight years of my life, eight years that would have been very important to me. They should have been formative years, and I was stuck in a bloody hospital' (Rhona). 'It's a nightmare isn't it? Honest to God I wake up in the middle of the night thinking about that operation and everything. And I keep thinking of all the horrible things that have happened' (Georgina). 'With this y'can't overcome it. No matter what you try. It keeps on knocking you down. I guess it's some kind of psychological thing, you lose confidence, and become anti-social' (Andrew). 'I do most of my thinking in bed. You lie and think, and it's the thought of having it for the rest of your life' (Pauline). 'I keep thinking "Why me? What did I do to deserve it?" I was never a drinker, I don't smoke, I don't gamble. I haven't smoked for twenty-odd years' (Bert).

For the subjects just quoted their feelings seemed to be of generalized unhappiness. For other respondents the problems seemed more deep seated. John, for example: 'It really hit me. This is not just like a broken leg that's going to heal in a few weeks' time. This is you for life. I was right depressed about it. I still am.' And Maggie, who said that at one time she was very disturbed: 'I thought I was going to have a complete breakdown. I'd wake up in the night shaking. I had to get up, I couldn't lie down. Everything passed through me every fifteen minutes and I'd have to go and empty my bag. I had to keep walking all the time. I walked up and down, in one room and out of the other. I just lit one cigarette after another, it was really frightening.'

These extracts do not suggest that these subjects are more depressed, anxious and unhappy than the population at large. Neither do these extracts reveal anything about the origins and causes of the long-term post-operative anxieties and worries. What they do demonstrate is that some respondents believe themselves to have been depressed, anxious and lonely because of their operation. Some continue to feel that way for a long time after surgery. Significantly, they themselves attribute the origins of their feelings to their operation and to having an ileostomy. They provide an interpretative framework to account for this state of affairs which uses the operation as the means of explanation. This is important because what they are doing is to account for their own feelings by means of an appeal to the unique or special nature of their identity, namely their ileostomy. The past experiences of illness and surgery provide an interpretative framework which makes sense of present experience. It is a means of appraisal and as such is itself a means of coping. The verbal account, or attribution, of depression, anxiety, or loneliness is a coping strategy aimed at dealing with genuinely experienced psychological unease. This is not to argue that depression is a response to surgery. It might be, but these data cannot demonstrate that. This investigation demonstrates first, that some ex-patients believe that depression is a response to surgery, and second, that that belief helps them make sense of their world and helps other people, in turn, make sense of the exhibited behaviour.

The verbal attribution of psychological distress and personal problems to the operation is but one specific example of a verbal coping device. Verbal coping devices were routinely used by respondents. They can take various forms and have differing content, but their purpose is twofold: to offer to the listener a particular version of self for acknowledgement and confirmation and to provide an interpretative framework both to reappraise past events and to furnish motives for future actions (cf. Mills, 1940).

A few examples serve to demonstrate the idea. In the first, identity develops out of an epic struggle, in which the respondent has successfully encountered the most adverse of circumstances and triumphed over them. Christine for example: 'It's never been a problem. There's nothing you can't do. And if you have a problem it can be solved. I always say that if I could go through that, bad as it was, there's nothing else ever going to be as bad again.' And Tom: 'I just take each day as it comes. It's not a nice thing to have but I'm healthy and fit again. I couldn't go back to what I was like before. It was a hell of a life, it was terrible. I've no regrets. I'd rather be normal but you must accept it, you must get on with life, it's as simple as that.'

In the next set of extracts the way the subjects were attempting to present themselves to the interviewer was in terms of being the victim of a tragedy in which the passage through illness and surgery was one of downfall from health. 'I used to think about it a lot. Why do you get it? What causes it? Why have I got it? What have I done to deserve this?' (Pauline). 'I mean okay having an ulcer taken out, that's an operation, bang! They stitch you up and that's you. But coming to terms with yourself, with the fact that you've got your bag on your side. If they hadn't operated it would have been the pine box for me' (Bert).

For some respondents there were lessons to be drawn from the experience, hidden benefits or personal growth. Annie said, 'I really have got a new lease of life since this. I have had a very good life, and I've never really been ill', and Julie said, 'In spite of being disfigured my husband says, "Its better having you here, because if you didn't have that bag you wouldn't be here." I look down and I think I'm glad they were able to do something for me. You think you are bad until you see other people, it makes you thankful.'

In each of these extracts the subjects have chosen to portray themselves in particular ways. They are offering an account of themselves as particular kinds of people who have survived surgery or been changed by surgery, because of who, or what sort of person they are. These data suggest that verbal accounting practices are important coping devices in themselves. While these accounts may or may not be a true representation of what 'really' happened, or what the subjects 'truly' felt, the accounts have an additional function in that they are a coping strategy in their own right. They help to preserve particular self-images and conceptions and present desirable identities. The account is an interpretative framework which is a means of appraisal of current events and a reappraisal of the past. It helps to make sense of things and it helps to explain things. The person is in effect saying, 'I coped the way I did because that is the kind of person I am and it was not unreasonable to behave in that way, given the circumstances.'

One important element in such accounts is the strong emphasis on the fact that post-operative life is better than pre-operative life. The subject produces an account in which pre-operative life was one in which the person was ill, had suffered, and whose life was in danger. These are considerable threats. The new post-operative life is one free of disease and of restriction, a life of mobility and activity and freedom from pain. The new life offers hope. The old life represents a negative identity, the new life a positive one. Where the individual's self-image and self-conception encapsulates these elements, and where the substantial identity is one of a well person, almost any discomfort associated with the ileostomy seems to be manageable. As Kathleen said, 'You see, I have looked and I have seen. I've had so much pain and discomfort before, that anything was going to be better. I reason that if I didn't have this I would have died of cancer.' And Melanie said, 'I have not looked back. I've certainly got no regrets about having it done. I haven't felt as healthy as this for some time. I haven't regretted it, and I'm leading a perfectly normal life now, which I feel I couldn't have done before.' Harry also pointed to the advantages. 'The transformation between what you can do now, what you can eat, the exercise you can do, the self-confidence you've got, compared with what you had beforehand is enormous. You couldn't participate in sports, anywhere you went you virtually had to have a route map of toilets and goodness knows what else, and severe dietary restrictions, so really it has been quite a transformation.'

Sally was another person who was very positive: 'I walk jauntily down the street, I couldn't have done that. Last Sunday I went for a stroll in the park. There's no way I could have done that before. As for thinking about going on holiday anywhere, that was quite out of the question. Oh it was a miserable existence. I have to admit that my surgeon was right when he said that he would change my life.' And finally Donna: 'I didn't have to think about the loo, or whether I will manage to get to it in time, not to be able to go shopping because there is no toilet there, I don't think about it now.'

Conclusion

An important sociological concept which has some bearing on the issues discussed in this chapter is that of stigma. In particular the distinction between discreditable and discredited stigma is helpful (Goffman, 1968). A discreditable stigma is some physical or moral negative aspect or attribute of a person implying inferiority and disgrace, which is not publicly known either by close intimates or by strangers. A discredited stigma, on the other hand, is one that is obvious, such as facial deformity or limb amputation. An ileostomy is a good example of a discreditable stigma in so far as it is not obvious, but when it becomes so, if it becomes so, it is likely to attract negative evaluations from others. A key problem for the person with an ileostomy, as was shown in this chapter, is physically that of managing the stoma, and socially that of managing the information about self in such a way that the ileostomy remains a potential but not actual stigma. It also shows that great skills, or a thick skin are required to brazen things out when leaks occur or when for other reasons the ileostomy becomes public knowledge (see also Scambler and Hopkins, 1986: 33).

Another important set of sociological ideas which are germane to the data reported here are the notions of primary and secondary deviation (Lemert, 1967: 40–1). Primary deviation from normality is a consequence of difference for an individual and it matters little whether the differences are social, psychological or physiological, and it matters still less what the cause of the difference is; it is the fact of difference which is important. The critical thing about primary deviation is that it has only marginal implications for the social status and the psychic structure of the individual who is different. Secondary deviation is also based on difference, but it occurs where there is a wholesale social reaction to the difference that has a profound effect on the person: the difference is no longer marginal, it becomes the central fact of existence for those involved, altering psychic structure, producing highly specialized social roles and attitudes. Life is organized around the facts of difference.

When someone has an operation that gives them an ileostomy, what first happens in sociological terms is secondary deviation; the whole life of the person revolves around the operation and its sequelae. Gradually however, if the ileostomy can be managed, concealed, and kept out of the gaze of the world at large, and the person goes back to leading a life of functioning ordinarily, then he or she is in a situation of primary deviation: his or her difference makes no difference. For the person with an ileostomy whose life remains forever locked into a central concern with the ileostomy, who never escapes from the tyranny of the difference, it is appropriate to think in terms of a life of secondary deviation. For still others, life oscillates between primary and secondary deviation as they remain more or less in control of their ileostomy, its appliance and indeed of themselves.

Overall, the main social-psychological process which the data have highlighted concern the tension in identity, between the normal and the normal-but-different identity. The person with an ileostomy appears to be normal when fully clothed, but underneath it all, the body works differently. Quite apart from coping with the ileostomy and its appliance, the person with an ileostomy has to cope with that social-psychological process. It is ultimately a tension between a biological contingency (the difference) and a social fact (the appearance of normality).

What the respondents' statements reported in this chapter point to, is that for people with an ileostomy the relationship between biological and social processes is important. They have a stoma which is a biological fact. They will be subjectively aware of this and a relatively small number of significant others will share that information. Outside that small circle they will appear to be quite ordinary and will be acted towards by others as if there were no ileostomy. This social fact of being treated in exactly the same way as anybody else, is, however, a contingent one. It depends upon coping mechanisms working, and it depends on the help or team-work of significant others who are 'in the know'.

Help or team work implies in a sociological sense, as Goffman reminded us, co-involvement, a common enemy, and rule governed interaction (Goffman, 1972: 31–8). The other side are those who are not in the know, and from whom it is necessary to conceal the true facts. The team can only relax, to borrow another of Goffman's metaphors, in backstage settings. Front stage is where apparent identities are sustained, managed and presented to audiences who are unaware of the biological facts. Backstage is the arena in which performances are prepared, precautions are taken, appliances made ready, and accidents cleaned up (Goffman, 1969). It is the private world hidden from wider view, shared with intimates and co-players, where the real person can be comfortably exposed and relaxation from the performance enjoyed. In many respects, just like Goffman's stage metaphor, backstage life for the person with an ileostomy may be chaotic and tense, involving much make-do-and-mend, like all theatres in real life as opposed to the sociological figure of speech.

People with an ileostomy have to work hard to sustain their appearance of ordinariness. Perhaps as the years go by and they become more experienced and technically proficient the work becomes easier, but work it is. It is an effortful process (Strauss et al., 1984). In order to make sense of all this, the elaborate accounting mechanisms and stories which these subjects told about themselves should also be noted. One of the ways of coping with the tensions and difficulties is talking about them in ways which provide particular verbal explanations of events. Coping is central to the life of the person with an ileostomy and linguistic practices are a cornerstone of the coping. This talk does not represent some other aspect of coping, it is itself part of coping.

Chapter six

The experience of colitis and colectomy

Coping with illness and surgery

In this chapter a model of coping is presented which is developed from the accounts in the previous chapters. The analysis begins with a further consideration of the ideas of self and identity. Throughout the book the term 'self' has referred to the idea of the individual's private view of who and what he or she is, while the term 'identity' has referred to the public view or perception that others have of the person. This distinction is helpful in understanding the situation of someone who has colitis or an ileostomy whose sense of self has to embrace the highly restricting nature of the symptoms as well as the altered sense of self contingent on the ileostomy. This private sense of difference is not a public announcement nor signifier of difference. Hence the public identity is 'normal' while the illness and the ileostomy are being coped with.

Selves and identities are both stable and changing. William James, the American philosopher, made this point when he wrote,

> If [in] the sentence 'I am the same as I was yesterday', we take the 'I' broadly, it is evident that in many ways I am *not* the same. As a concrete Me, I am somewhat different from what I was: then hungry, now full; then walking, now at rest; then poorer, now richer; then younger, now older; etc. And yet in other ways I *am* the same, and we may call these the essential ways. My name and profession and relations to the world are identical, my face, my faculties and store of memories are practically indistinguishable, now and then. Moreover, the Me of now and the Me of then are *continuous*.
>
> (James, 1968: 47)

More recently the American social psychologist Turner has

expressed the same idea. Turner distinguishes between self-image and self-conception. Self-image is that which is tied to particular situations or contexts. This is the snapshot, the picture in the individual's mind's eye of the 'real me'. Self-image can change from moment to moment and may be diverse and multiple, depending on the various audiences the person imagines himself or herself to be addressing. The snapshot also may be false, unrepresentative or misguided. Self-conception, on the other hand, changes more slowly. It is more coherent and is linked to the social structure because it represents the way people see themselves as fitting in with the broader social world around them (Turner, 1968: 94). The self, for the purposes of the model developed in this chapter is taken to be both variable and stable (Rosenberg, 1981: 593–4), it is continuous but it is also changing, it is holistic and it is fragmented (Stone and Farberman, 1970; Rosenberg, 1981: 593–4).

Similarly identities are neither permanent nor fixed, nor entirely situationally determined. Identities emerge in social situations, but are not determined by social situations. Once having emerged they may become powerful determinants of the social structure in the form of stable social roles. Identities and selves may have an enduring, lasting quality across time and situation.

Four conceptual categories are therefore identifiable in respect of self and identity, and reflect change and permanence: self-image, which is the situationally specific element concerned with the here and now; self-concept, which is concerned with the enduring features of selfhood; situated identity, which is those aspects of identity which are situationally specific and concerned with the here and now; and substantial identity, which is concerned with the stable, long-term enduring aspects of identity (Ball, 1972).

Coping

In both common-sense usage and in scientific writings about it, the term 'coping' is used in two different and overlapping ways. There is the use of coping to mean 'getting on top of' or mastering events, or control of circumstances. Coping is also used as a synonym for adjustment or accommodation; it refers to dealing with anything and everything, great or small. The former usage tends to refer to the extraordinary, sudden and unanticipated major and acute events with which people have to cope (for example, sudden bereavement, disaster, acute illness, personal tragedy), while the latter usage tends to refer to longer-term continuous aggravating major and minor consistent and chronic difficulties (for example, straitened economic circumstances, unhappy relationships, long-term illness). A model of coping has to embrace both meanings of the term. Linking the ideas of change and continuity to self and identity provides this facility.

It is also worth noting that both in common-sense use and in some of the scientific literature concerned with coping, there is the ascription of positive or negative values to certain types of coping actions. Some coping behaviour is seen as good because it has beneficial or adaptive outcomes, while other coping behaviour is seen as ineffective or maladaptive and therefore bad. The problem with this is twofold; the emphasis on the outcome of the behaviour rather than the behaviour itself is a rather static way of conceptualizing human conduct; and if we are to pass judgement on how well or badly someone coped, it must be very clearly understood precisely whose values are being used as the yardstick – those of the coper or of the observer. The concepts of self and identity allow for a plurality of judgements about the coping behaviour.

The literature, especially the psychological literature, dealing with coping is massive, and it would be inappropriate in a text of this type to attempt a comprehensive review (but see Kelly, 1990). Four elements in the literature must, however, be emphasized. First, there is a considerable body of work where the focus is almost exclusively on psychological processes within individuals. Thus coping has been described as a technique for mastering psychological threat and its attendant negative feelings (Mattson, 1977: 183–99; Moos and Tsu, 1977: 9) and for resolving anxiety and psychological distress (Myers et al., 1977: 224; Tropauer et al., 1977: 212; Bieliaukas, 1982). Explanations of outcomes of coping have been linked to pre-traumatic personality (Visotsky et al., 1961: 424; Lipowski, 1970: 93–100), psychodynamic regression (Abram, 1970; Adler, 1972) and self-concepts (Simmons et al., 1985: 111). Haan, approaching the issue from a psychoanalytic perspective, argued that the inner self is critical in understanding coping. Coping, she suggested, is concerned with a person's inner phenomenology and attempts to make self-consistent sense out of self and what others and the world make of self (Haan, 1977: 2). Dealing with stressful encounters involves, for Haan, protection of intra-subjective valuation which in its turn, is about the transaction with external valuation of self by others (1977: 192). The concept of self may be used to elaborate these individualistic types of processes.

Second, there are a number of writers who have attended to the person–person and person–environment aspects of coping, defining it as a social behaviour, rather than as a psychological process *per se*. Seligman, for example, linked coping with mastery, as against helplessness in the environment (Seligman, 1975: 55), while Visotsky *et al.* (1961), Walker *et al.* (1977), and New *et al.* (1968: 195) underline, in different ways, and circumstances, the great importance of supportive social relationships with other people, and what are called in the literature social networks, in coping. The concept of identity helps to embrace the inter-personal aspect of coping.

The third strand in the literature is concerned with the scope of coping. Some authors have analysed coping in the face of extreme events. Exceptional and dramatic crises are highlighted and attention is drawn to the strain put upon individuals under such circumstances. The classical approach in this vein deals with responses to disasters (see especially Lindemann, 1944). Other writers have emphasized the very ordinary, routine and unexceptional nature of coping (see, for example, Pearlin, 1985). Writers such as Pearlin tend to see life as intrinsically difficult in an all embracing sense, rather than consisting of periods of peace and tranquillity disrupted by disasters that need to be coped with. For Pearlin, to live is to cope. The ideas of continuity and change, already alluded to, allow the description of both the ordinary and the exceptional.

The last general point about the literature which deals with coping is the concern with the thing that has to be coped with. There is widespread agreement that one of the problems bedevilling research that sought biological or psychological responses to 'stressors' was isolating the cause of stress. What was a stressor to one person or animal, would not invariably be a source of stress to another person or animal, and the same object, or 'stressor' would not always produce stress even in the same person or animal. The process of interpretation of the environment and the ability to discriminate between objects which are dangerous or threatening and those which are not is an absolutely and fundamental part of coping. Lazarus's work, which has informed the analysis in this book, has been seminal in drawing attention to the processes of appraisal (primary and secondary) which are concerned with discrimination and interpretation of the environment (Lazarus, 1976; see also Janis and Mann, 1977).

The four elements which have informed social scientific research on coping form the basis of the model of coping developed here. These are:

1 That individual psychological processes are highly important because there is often massive and emotional involvement in the events which have to be coped with.
2 That coping takes place in a social and inter-personal environment which constrains and facilitates coping.
3 That coping has to be understood both as a behaviour taking place in the face of massively disruptive life events as well as a behaviour which is routinely used in the most mundane of circumstances.
4 That predicting the triggers of coping is problematic because the origin of stress is not a property of the external object but a property of the interpreting subject, it is a question of meaning.

Self is concerned principally with psychological processes, whereas identity is about the social processes. The ideas of change and permanence are also involved because of the concern with cataclysmic change, and major life events. This is embraced in the concepts of situational identity and self-image, while the routine permanent nature of coping is captured in the more enduring ideas of self-concept and substantial identity (Ball, 1972). Meaning and processes of appraisal develop in the interchange between the self and others and in the creation and negotiation of identity.

It will now be argued that self-image and self-concept and situated and substantial identity provide a means of theorizing coping with chronic illness and debilitating surgery.

Ways and means of coping

When the illness ulcerative colitis first begins, most coping behaviour is concerned with self-image. The person's normal sense of self is violated and initially nearly all the coping is private and self-oriented. When the disease appears it is not generally recognized as a disease. Prospective patients do at some point observe a deviation in their bowel habit, but the typical response of the people interviewed in this study was to define such deviations as irrelevant, benign or as within the range of normal experience. These are not unreasonable things to do given that diarrhoea and even pain are not unusual and, as such, can be routinely coped with by doing nothing very much. However, the symptoms of ulcerative colitis can be insistent and the appearance of blood often signals a need for the individual to revise his or her initial hypothesis. To this point the coping is *intra-subjective*. It involves thought processes, appraisals and evaluations, and operates at the level of psychological processing and intellectual reasoning. The person brings to bear knowledge and attitudes which are culturally derived and socially learned, but interactive behaviours as such are minimal.

At the point at which the person translates self-indicated deviations from bodily normality into a problem which significantly interferes with desired or required activities, or at the point at which benign symptoms are reappraised as highly threatening, for example because of the appearance of blood, a change in self-image occurs in which seeking out help is deemed to be legitimate. The behaviour ceases to be entirely at the psychological level and at once becomes *inter-personal*, and therefore issues of identity are raised.

Seeking help, it was shown, could take a number of forms, either medical, alternative medical, non-medical or all three. Interaction with others is involved and through a sometimes lengthy process, the medical profession assumes a key role. In western society, the fact that medical help-seeking is a routine coping behaviour is scarcely a surprising finding. Thus far the description of coping would be exactly as predicted by such writers as Parsons (1951), Mechanic (1962), and Zola (1965).

Once these proto-patients initiate contact with the medical profession this opens up a new range of problems which themselves have to be coped with, in addition to the ongoing symptoms. For some people initial contact with the GP not only does *not* lead to a diagnosis but is met with a denial of the seriousness of the problem by the physician. The person's hypothesis that he or she has something wrong which is serious enough to warrant seeing a doctor, is dismissed.

If symptoms remit, this is not a problem. However, symptoms may worsen and proto-patients find themselves coping with the denial of their sensory experience by their doctor. The coping actions seen in this book include a determination to try and convince the doctor, or perhaps trying to find a different doctor. The sheer happenstance of the availability of particular GPs, their locums, their partners, was an important variable to some extent independent of symptoms, which determined the speed at which diagnosis was made. The proto-patient has to cope both with their symptoms and a primary care system. That which should alleviate the problem becomes part of the problem. The patient response may well be to consult 'inappropriate' non-medical or alternative medical advisers as well as attempts to 'educate' their own physicians.

However, not all patients face this problem, and for many, medical advisers recognize the legitimacy of their behaviour in seeking medical help and the process of diagnosis begins. Diagnosis is highly significant in the process of coping because it is linked to the questions of appraisal and meaning. Diagnosis leads to treatment; diagnosis also confirms the legitimacy of the actions of the patient in having sought help in the first place. But in terms of coping, the diagnosis also provides a disease label which is a conceptual framework for appraising past actions and future options.

Going to see a doctor is a type of *inter-personal* behaviour. It involves acquiring a particular kind of identity, that of patient. This is a situated identity locked closely into the context of the initial symptoms, the immediate pain and discomfort and the difficulties and problems associated with the illness. It is a situated identity because, by and large, it is viewed as a temporary or passing state of affairs. The patient envisages a future when he or she will be well again. Acquiring a diagnosis is, amongst other things, about acquiring meaning. In social-psychological, as opposed to medico-scientific terms, the diagnosis provides the patient with a shared or an *inter-subjective* theory with which to interpret the experience. In the hands of the patient the diagnosis is an accounting framework. It is a symbolically powerful inter-subjective category which the patient has earned or acquired the right to use. For a lay person the diagnostic label provides the means of analysing the threat and danger associated with the symptoms and for deciding what may be done about them. This is not to say that patients use diagnostic categories in the same way that doctors do. Patients may comply with their medical treatment on the basis of their doctor's diagnosis, but equally, they may resist or ignore the efforts of their medical helpers. Such resistance may be purely cognitive (the patient may be doubtful or sceptical). Alternatively resistance may be behavioural and treatments may be avoided and appointments missed.

Diagnosis may itself be viewed as a threat by the patient, especially where the provision of the disease label ends an uncertainty which patients may have invested effort and time in encouraging. Sometimes patients have developed very strong attachments to being ill, but undiagnosable. The threat is to the benefits of having a mystery illness. However, much the most common reaction was for diagnosis to be a source of relief.

In focusing on self-image and situated identity as the symptoms are first noticed and then diagnosed and as the patient comes into the orbit of medical practice, three types of coping may be highlighted. First, a set of coping activities which are principally psychological or *intra-subjective*; second, a set of *inter-personal* transactions; and third, a process of rendering what has happened as meaningful using *inter-subjective* categories.

During the progress of the illness into a chronic course, a range of other behaviours was observed. It was noted that one habitual coping device was the incorporation of symptom experience into routine experience. The sense of self changes. The constancy of the symptoms and their ubiquitous accompaniment to everyday activities has an associated process of internal psychological activity which, because of its habitual nature, becomes second nature. Symptoms become the background to living and as background are appraised, not as benign, but as something about which little can be done. This is marked even in the case of pain. For some respondents pain was defined as irrelevant and something about which the medical profession was capable of doing very little.

However, coping routinely with the disease is not only a psychological process. The unpredictability of bowel function cannot itself be controlled by wishful thinking and episodes of public self-soiling or the threat of that self-soiling, cannot easily be defined as irrelevant. It was observed that some, perhaps a majority of patients, therefore develop two types of skill: constantly scanning the environment for escape routes and developing highly detailed knowledge about the whereabouts of usable toilets. They also develop appropriate exit lines (physical and verbal). That skill also involves the habitual planning of activities in order to allow for a semblance of normal functioning. The critical task is of presenting a normal identity and of maintaining the appearance of normality, in contrast to the self-concept which has to embrace the disease. Sufferers have to alter their own view of who and what they are, while attempting more or less to preserve a substantial identity as ordinary people. Given the episodic nature of the illness and the skills which they develop, this may be a highly effective strategy and only a few intimates may know what the true situation is. On the other hand if symptoms are highly intrusive, if the person is bedridden and debilitated, any semblance of a public identity as someone who is well is clearly out of the question.

The person with colitis faces a tension between the demands made by their illness and the demands made by his or her normal role obligations. This is a common enough problem for any ill person, and indeed competing role obligations are part of normal human experience in health as well as sickness. The difference here is that the demands of the colitis may be kept secret by the sufferer and the compelling nature of the demands may be shared with only a few others: it is the attempt to carry on as if there were no illness which may be the complicating coping task. In this respect the patient is in analogous position to any human actor who wishes to keep some aspect of his or her self away from the gaze of the world at large. The ever present possibility of symptoms swamping social interaction gives an added dimension to the problem.

It was noted above that, because of their attempt to maintain a veneer of normality, subjects described their behaviour as 'carrying on regardless'. It was also observed that 'carrying on regardless' was not cost-free. Some people found it stressful in itself, certainly at times of acute exacerbation of the illness. Others withdrew from some types of high-risk activity like travel. Some introduced dietary restrictions. Some simply withdrew from some or all normal role obligations.

For still others, the illness represented a challenge which was to be fought back against. The distinction between carrying on regardless and fighting back is a fine one and many people seem to do both things. Carrying on regardless involved wilful ignoring of the problems caused by the symptoms, whereas fighting back involved a recognition of particular limitations and acting accordingly. In the face of these problems it was noted that respondents typically engaged in a process of appraisal or theorizing about their illness, frequently drawing upon the diagnostic framework and sometimes attempting to gather medical and pseudo-medical information about their complaint.

In terms of inter-personal relationships during illness, two rather distinct sets of coping issues face the individual. First, with non-significant others the effort is towards presenting normality in interaction and passing-off self as normal. The strategies which the ill person devises to do this are self-driven. It is the secrecy of the illness and the maintenance of that secrecy which means that non-significant others are not involved in a process of legitimating anything other than a normal version of self. Normal adult identity is maintained, or at least striven for, and this is the coping task, with the sub-routines of carrying on regardless, planning, scanning, fighting back and withdrawal.

This is not, however, something which can be achieved alone. In relationships with significant others, those significant others are drawn into the management of illness in order that a life of any kind beyond the immediate family might be sustained. The substantial identity which is created within the closed interaction with significant others is of normal-but-ill. That is, the person with colitis is more or less openly acknowledged in the family as someone who to all intents and purposes is normal, but who has a set of associated characteristics which have to be managed. This is coping in two ways; it underpins activities which allow the person to cope in interaction beyond the family or circle of intimate acquaintances, and it is a way of coping realistically with the problems generated by the symptoms within the private sphere of family life.

It was noted that the subjects in this study reported using collusive routines like closely controlling information, deliberately disregarding public manifestations of symptoms or the social behaviour associated with them. Sometimes other family members were reported as having markedly altered their own behaviour in order to help maintain the normal public identity of the sick person. It was also observed that collusive routines sometimes fail. This tended to happen either because people beyond the family circle refused to collaborate – this particularly being so in large-scale bureaucracies and employing organizations; it may also happen if family members stop playing the game. In these circumstances the only option then available to the person with the disease is withdrawal.

Medical consultations can be an important threat to successful coping as far as normal-but-ill identities are concerned. Being normal-but-ill does not fit with the rationale of some out-patient consultations, or at least may be perceived that way by the patient.

Consequently, because of the threat to the coping strategy some respondents seem to engage in highly negative stereotyping of their doctors. This seems to be particularly pronounced if the patient has already been informed that the condition is treatable only with surgery. The prospective threat of the operation highlights the ultimate failure, not only of medical treatment, but also of the coping via the normal-but-ill identity.

It is convenient to conceptualize coping with the illness at four levels: an *intra-subjective* or cognitive level; a level concerned with *skills* and their use in the practicalities of the illness; a level concerned with *inter-personal* relations, and a level which is *inter-subjective*, that is, concerned with the generation of meaning as public substantial identities are negotiated and sustained or rejected. Within the range of public identities for different audiences, the meaning which is generated may be variously normal, normal-but-ill, carrying on regardless, fighting back, victim of circumstances and so on; indeed there are a whole repertoire of appropriate categories. Where meaning cannot be negotiated, and where identity cannot be agreed, the coping activity of the ill person may be completely undermined.

When the prospect of surgery has to be confronted, the relatively stable routines for dealing with the illness may be overturned. The prospect of surgery is a new and mostly alarming prospect, which generates self-image and situated identity problems. A number of different reactions follow after learning of the prospect of surgery. Resistance to surgery may be the first reaction, as the patient possibly refuses to accept the prognosis or psychologically blocks out information. Alternatively some people take comfort in gathering as much information as they can about their medical condition. Still others invent reasons not to go to the hospital. These types of resistance behaviours may be rather half-hearted but they may continue up to the last minute before surgery.

The acceptance of surgery is not really a positive decision taken at a particular point in time. The decision is taken during a period of time which is a zone of transition in identity and self. Zones of transition may be short or long. Where they are short they are linked directly to the somatic course of the disease. Decline in health is great and being sick overrides any attempt to normalize the symptoms. Rational acceptance of the medical definition of the situation is seen as undesirable but logical and necessary, and the appraisal of the threat of surgery is weighed against the even greater threat from the disease. Where the zone of transition is lengthy and symptoms and their meaning more equivocal, those with colitis (and their significant others) may engage episodically in a complicated process of appraisal of the costs and benefits of the disease, as against surgery. This episodic process may be cyclical, involving subsequent and frequent reappraisals, especially during contact with medical advisers who may be urging surgery.

The experience of surgery itself creates very specific self-image issues and very particular situational identities as a sick person, as an acutely ill post-operative case, and as a recovering surgical patient. Going into hospital for colectomy involves a process of loss of self-control. These losses are reinforced by organizational factors in ward and hospital settings. Although some patients may try to fight back against organizational and medical imperatives, for many, the post-operative experience is one of feelings of loss of self and depersonalization. These acute experiences seem only to be resolved after the experience of intense anger or of doing 'grief work'. Even for those patients who did not report undergoing emotional trauma, being a surgical patient presents particular coping problems.

Surgical wards are organized inter-personally in ways both to encourage and to discourage dependence by patients on staff. They require total submission and then activity in search of convalescence (at least for this type of surgery). The organizational cues are ambiguous and therefore any appraisal process by the patient is difficult. Residual post-operative and drug effects can make active coping extremely complex. Coping with the new ileostomy under such circumstances is something which many respondents in this study seemed to slough off to their nurses and the process of learning to live with the ileostomy began only on discharge from hospital.

In terms of levels of coping and in terms of self-image and situational identity three elements can be identified: first, the *intra-subjective* or psychological element, which is the focus of the extreme emotions attaching to surgery, as well as the subjective decision-making process or zone of transition as the individual's self-image changes from that of someone who does not need surgery to someone who does; second, the *inter-personal* element involving situational identities, and in particular the intensely affective relationships in the wards between the patients and the nurses; third, the *inter-subjective* or meaning element, reflecting how the respondents make sense of what has happened to them and the point at which they think in terms of having 'come through' the experience.

The fourth element of coping, that concerned with basic skills to deal with the practicalities of having an ileostomy, comes later and relates to the development of stable self-concepts and substantial identities in the longer-term post-operative period. The *acquisition of skills* associated with the technical functioning of the ileostomy and its appliance are basic to the normal-but-different self-concept and the normal public substantial identity. Indeed so long as the ileostomy functions properly and there are no appliance problems then a pain-free and disease-free life are perfectly possible. To cope with a normally functioning ileostomy requires only that the now ex-patient follows very limited and not very limiting toileting and changing procedures. The most taxing task is keeping the appliance hidden.

However, in general terms, living with an ileostomy is not as simple as that. Problems crop up including stomal malfunction, appliance failure, and skin deterioration. Routine coping mechanisms will be habitually brought into play, such as regular changing, dietary discretion, anticipating problems, seeking medical help, and self-treatment. Occasionally, withdrawal into the sick role temporarily or permanently may be the action which is deployed.

Inter-personal intimate and sexual relationships constitute a particular problem. A prominent coping activity among the people interviewed in this study was the use of the ileostomy as a device to explain away difficulties in sexual relationships. Some people with ileostomies define their ileostomy as irrelevant in sexual encounters; this seems especially so among those in long-standing, well-established sexual relationships. Other people seem to avoid sexual contact altogether.

In inter-personal relations, people with an ileostomy can exert some degree of control over the information about themselves which they disclose to other people. Many seem to say nothing, act normally and indeed in most situations this is a highly effective and appropriate strategy. Other ileostomists selectively choose to reveal the fact that they have a stoma when there is no need for them to do so. Some seem to receive ego-satisfying rewards from this.

Finally, some of the people interviewed here reported feeling anger, depression and loneliness and attributed these feelings to their history of surgery or to the presence of the stoma. The stoma and the total experience of illness and surgery provide a wide-ranging interpretative framework which helps to make sense of things. This is critical in the generation of meaning. Strong elements concerning the benefits of post-operative life, compared to previous experience, figure in some coping accounts.

Once again a fourfold structure of the coping process can be highlighted. The first element is the *intra-subjective* or cognitive, and involves the thought processes and feelings, the anger, depression, loneliness and sadness. The second element is the *technical* with its concerns with the basic hand skills for manipulating and successfully using and wearing an appliance, as well as the necessary skills to use when malfunctions or minor or major complications occur. Third, the *inter-personal* element concerns the ways of dealing with intimates and non-intimates and in particular the management of information. Fourth, the *inter-subjective* element concerns accounts of the experiences which are themselves used as interpretative and sense-making devices (Kelly, 1991).

Conclusion: a sociology of coping with chronic illness

This study of the way people experience ulcerative colitis and total colectomy and ileostomy suggests that to experience the illness and its surgical sequelae involve four different behavioural components: the intra-subjective, the technical, the inter-personal and the inter-subjective. These four components transcend psychological and social factors.

The first component is the intra-subjective dimension; this is the thinking, feeling and emotional element of the experience of illness. It is the level of self-experience, of self-image changes in the face of altering circumstances and in self-conception in the case of more long-term concerns. It is the seat of pain and discomfort and the focus of the various mechanisms of the preservation of self and of psychological defence. It is that component of human experience that is sometimes called attitudes. This is not the determinant nor driver of behaviour but rather the starting-point of human conduct. It is the aspect of the person concerned with cognitive processes.

The second component is skill-based, and is principally technical or practical in orientation. Skills may take the form of particular hand skills such as changing and fixing an appliance, or they may be information based such as the knowledge of the whereabouts of toilet facilities or private changing rooms. The skills may relate to the routine taking of medication during the illness, the self-administration of enemas or any of the many anti-pollution routines in bedrooms, bathrooms and other places, where the person with colitis has to clean up after self-soiling. The technical skills are primarily body management ones designed to curtail the outflow of waste from the body, either during the illness or once the ileostomy is *in situ*. Without these technical skills, other routine social intercourse is impossible, because it is they which hold the biological contingency of the illness in check. As with all skills they are acquired, so when people first become ill with ulcerative colitis, or when they first have their ileostomy they do not have the technical skills with which to cope and they have many more accidents. Thus, these skills are part of the more stable self-concept, they are a means of sustaining self against the travails of the illness and the surgery.

The third component is concerned with inter-personal interactions. It is about physical action in space and time. It is that aspect of coping that occurs when the thinking human actor meets other thinking human actors. It takes place in, and is constrained by organizational and environmental contexts. It is concerned with identities; it is where situational identities are negotiated and generated and it is the setting in which substantial identities interleave with social behaviour.

The fourth component is verbal, and is concerned with meaning. It is the manner and way in which actors account for, explain and justify what they have done in the past, what they are doing now and what they will do in the future. Such verbal behaviours are common-sense inter-subjective categories like disease labels and models of cause and effect and contain elements of narrative as part of their interpretative armoury. These categories are inter-subjectively shared, or at least are taken as shared by their users. Because of their assumed inter-subjectivity they constitute part of the world of public discourse – as against the private rather incohate experiences of emotion, anger, and depression which constitute the intra-subjective level. These verbalizations have the quality of scientific theories, although they are of course lay theories. They attempt to answer such questions as why? how?. what? when? and where? These accounts both impute or attribute cause (justification) and demonstrate it (explanation, rationalization). Clearly such verbal theorizing and accounting feed back to the intra-subjective aspect and for all practical rather than analytic purposes, are difficult to separate from it. The more deep rooted and routinized they become, the greater role they play in respect of substantial identity and stable self-concept (cf. Mills, 1940; Schutz, 1967).

Over the years the kinds of behaviours which have been described in this study have attracted the attention of sociologists, psychologists and others who have been interested in responses to chronic illness. Terms such as denial, attenuation, resignation, normalization and so on have been used to describe the processes concerned. Denial, for example, as a response to illness has been described by Lipowski (1969: 1202), Moss (1972: 12), Zola (1982: 84), and Moos and Tsu (1977: 13, 97–8), among many. Denial, seen either as a mechanism of psychological defence or as an irrational response to the illness, would be a way to describe some of the behaviours reported in this text. Recast in terms of the model of coping developed in this study, denial may be conceptualized as the process whereby self denies or refuses to acknowledge the disease at a cognitive or intra-subjective level (the disease is not part of the self-image), while the situational identity bestowed by others at the inter-personal level is one of sick person. Because of the disjunction between the intra-subjective and inter-personal level, denial is inherently unstable. It requires verbal reparation by self or others to explain away the disjunction or to convince self or others of the 'true' state of affairs. At the intra-subjective level ego proclaims 'I am not sick'. Technically ego possesses no skills to handle being ill other than to deny. At the inter-personal level a sick identity is constructed by doctors, employers, family or other significant people. At the inter-subjective level some attempt has to be made to account for what is happening. This pattern is fairly typical of initial reactions to the illness. Rather than perceiving denial in these circumstances as evidence of a malformed psyche incapable of dealing with reality or as an automatic psychological defence, it is better to regard it a *realistic* response in the absence of the necessary skills to deal with the illness. Once other skills are learned and the illness can be incorporated into the more stable self-concept, denial probably features less prominently as a coping strategy or a response to illness. It may occur again when some new problem has to be dealt with (like surgery, in these cases) but its role will be less important.

Attenuation and avoidance are terms also to be found in the literature dealing with response to illness. Broadly, these two terms refer to strategies which involve the reduction of the significance of symptoms in various ways (see, for example, Visotsky *et al.*, 1961; Davis, 1963; Kosa and Robertson, 1969; Lipowski, 1970; Fager-haugh, 1973; Reif, 1973a and 1973b; Wiener, 1975; West, 1976). These strategies can vary from self-imposed social restrictions (Fagerhaugh, 1973: 95; MacDonald *et al.*, 1982: 89) to controlling information (White *et al.*, 1948: 20; Moos and Tsu, 1977: 14). In terms of the model of coping developed in this study, attenuation involves a recognition by self, at the intra-subjective level, that the body is diseased (it is part of stable self-conception) and self admits and recognizes that the disease presents problems. Public identity at the inter-personal level, on the other hand, while being explicitly associated with being sick, is not totally embraced by or stigmatized by the disease. The sickness or disease is not the master status or defining characteristic of the person. It is part of the acknowledged identity of the actor, but only a part of that acknowledged identity. At the technical skill level, coping involves very careful impression management in order to compensate for the negative aspects of identity, and a range of illness-related technical skills operate in order to maintain something like normal functioning. At the inter-subjective level a range of verbal categories are used in talk which not infrequently contain notions of fighter or victim. If the skills and impression management are sufficiently competent it may only be necessary for the public identity of the sick person to be known to a very few other people. In these circumstances social context and the nature of the players in the interaction will be critical in understanding the development of particular strategies. From the point of view of self, attenuation and avoidance involve a realistic acceptance of the limitations and difficulties which the disease presents, taking certain active technical steps to deal with those limitations and difficulties (without denying their importance) and behaving accordingly. The responses of others depend on their inside knowledge and extent of collusion with the sick person. Others who cease to collude have the potential to destroy the coping response (a difficult employer or partner has this potential, for example). These strategies are biologically contingent, because if symptoms intrude to any great extent, the strategy will disintegrate anyway.

Normalizing is a term that often crops up in the literature and is usually, but not invariably used to refer to the redefinition of deviance associated with the illness. Thus Zola uses the term to mean the reconstruction of discomfort as non-threatening (1982: 205) while Davis argues that normalizing means that those aspects of the person which distinguish and cause him or her to be different from normal, are made light of and rationalized away (Davis, 1963: 139–40). Normalizing has also been used to refer to acting 'as if' normal (Wiener, 1975: 99). The strategy involves an acknowledgement at the intra-subjective level that the changes (which medically are symptomatic of a particular illness) really exist as self-indicated phenomena, but that these changes are not symptoms of an illness, but rather are part of normal experience. In accounting terms, at the inter-subjective level it requires a redefinition of what is normal. Inter-personally these redefinitions are, tacitly at least, not challenged. It is very important that others reciprocate the redefinitions of things, otherwise the strategy cannot succeed. If familiar social contexts change, normalizing strategies will be under threat too.

Disavowal and passing are two terms frequently associated with responses to chronic illness. Passing is defined by Davis as the acceptance of normal standards and the desire to be viewed in terms of them and consequently eradicating and disguising the illness or disability (Davis, 1963: 138; Scambler and Hopkins, 1986: 33; West, 1985: 114–20). In terms of the present model of coping this type of behaviour works as follows. At the intra-subjective level, self acknowledges the fact of unusual body experiences as symptoms of illness (it is part of stable self-conception), but at the inter-personal level behaviour patterns do not reveal the presence of the disease or symptoms, and an identity is constructed of a healthy person. At the inter-subjective level the person proclaims health, and indeed may very well deny the illness itself, if asked directly. Other people are therefore not routinely privy to the knowledge of the condition. This type of behaviour tends to be premised on the view that if the true nature of self is revealed then a negative and stigmatizing label will be forthcoming. The success or otherwise of such strategies will depend on skilful competence in role performance and associated activities in bringing off normal identity. In many social situations passing and disavowal are not only highly appropriate, they allow routine interaction to proceed uninterrupted by the burden of illness. Although there are elements of deception involved, it would be wrong to think of these behaviours as fundamentally dishonest since most of the time the deception works in everybody's interest.

Accommodation to illness and resignation to illness are the last two concepts worth drawing from the more general literature on chronic illness. Accommodation is conventionally used to refer to a 'well-adjusted' patient (Lipowski, 1970: 97; Herzlich, 1973: 119; D'Afflitti and Weitz, 1977: 138–9) whereas resignation usually refers to someone who is completely overwhelmed by his or her disease (Chodoff, 1959: 663; Engel, 1968: 294; Eardley, 1977: 388). By implication accommodation and its variants are seen as good and resignation as bad. In fact, in terms of the coping model developed here they are really two sides of the same coin. Accommodation is the process whereby at the intra-subjective, technical, inter-personal and inter-subjective levels there is a consistent message which is that the illness is an important, stable and enduring part of the person (parts of self-conception and substantial identity) and is a characteristic of the person of which due account must be taken. However, the illness is not *the* most important aspect of the person and other social, psychological, economic political, religious or other variants of the human condition are presented as more important. Self wants to engage with the world not as a sick person, but someone who is *x*, *y* or *z* (and who also happens to be ill).

In contrast, resignation is the process whereby at the intra-subjective, technical, inter-personal and inter-subjective levels there is a consistent message which is that the most and only really important thing about the person is the fact that he or she is ill, and the only way the person engages with the world is on those terms. In response, the identity which the world bestows is of sick person. The self-conception and substantial identity are entirely wrapped up in illness. In accommodation the individual is a person who *has* ulcerative colitis or *has* an ileostomy. In resignation the person *is* a colitic or *is* an ileostomist.

The importance of examining briefly the concepts of normalizing, attenuation, resignation and the others and demonstrating their structure in terms of the fourfold model of coping is to make a plea for coping to be seen as an all embracing social process which operates at four distinct behavioural levels and not as an individualistic trait. The danger with discrete concepts like normalizing, denial and so on, is that they can so easily be represented as traits residing in individuals and the scientific task in understanding the experience of illness becomes one of identifying the various social and or psychological factors which will allow for prediction as to which person will be a denier, a resigner, and an accommodator. It is not a great step then to move into a kind of quasi-epidemiology of coping, which seeks to identify the percentage of sufferers with a particular disease who are deniers, the percentage who are accommodators and so on.

The experience of illness as opposed to the social epidemiology of disease is not really like that. The model of coping developed here does not allow for prediction as to who will cope well or who will cope badly. Its message is at once more subtle and more obvious. When people cope they use a *range* of strategies. Perhaps when they are first ill, or when they first develop symptoms they deny things; perhaps when acutely ill they resign themselves to their illness; perhaps when their symptoms are under control they will be accommodators. The fact is that the experience of illness is of the use of different strategies at different times. People who have a long chronic illness will run the gauntlet of these strategies as they think fit, as social circumstances suggest and as social interaction allows. They operate on the four levels here described and the process of their experience of coping with the illness will reflect the repertoires, skills, social circumstances, social intimates and social and economic resources available to them. To live is to cope, and to be ill is to cope. However, coping is not a trait, a style, nor an outcome; it is a social-psychological process which operates at four analytically distinct levels and which manifests itself in the range of behaviours described in this book. The experience of illness is the experience of coping with illness. Commonsensically the man or woman in the street knows that; social-psychologically this text has attempted to demonstrate how that works.

References

Abram, H.S. (1970) 'Survival by machine: the psychological stress of chronic hemodialysis', *Psychiatry in Medicine*, 1: 37–51.

Adler, M.L. (1972) 'Kidney transplantation and coping mechanisms', *Psychosomatics*, 13: 337–41.

Allan, H. and Hodgson, H. (1986) 'Inflammatory bowel disease', in Pounder, R. (ed.) *Recent Advances in Gastroenterology*, Churchill Livingstone, Edinburgh.

Andrew, J. (1970) 'Recovery from surgery with or without preparatory instruction for three coping styles', *Journal of Personality and Social Psychology*, 15: 223–6.

Ball, D. (1972) 'Self and identity in the context of deviance: the case of criminal abortion', in Scott, R.A. and Douglas, J.D. (eds) *Theoretical Perspectives on Deviance*, Basic Books, New York.

Bieliaukas, L. (1982) *Stress and its Relationship to Health and Illness*, Westview Press, Boulder, Colorado.

Binder, V., Weeke, E., Olsen, J., Anthonisen, P. and Riis, P. (1966) 'A genetic study of ulcerative colitis', *Scandanavian Journal of Gastroenterology*, 1: 49–56.

Bouchier, I. (1977) *Gastroenterology*, Balliere Tindall, London.

Brooke, B. (1986) *The Troubled Gut: The Causes and Consequences of Diarrhoea*, King Edward's Hospital Fund for London, London.

Burke, P. (1980) 'The self: measurement requirements from an interactionist perspective', *Social Psychology Quarterly*, 43: 18–29.

Bury, M. (1982) 'Chronic disease as biographical disruption', *Sociology of Health and Illness*, 4: 167–82.

Caplan, G. (1964) *Principles of Preventive Psychiatry*, Tavistock, London.

Charmaz, K. (1987) 'Struggling for a self: identity levels of the chronically ill', in Roth, J. and Conrad, P. (eds) *The Experience and Management of Chronic Illness: Research in the Sociology of Health Care*, Vol. 6, JAI Press, Greenwich, Connecticut.

Chodoff, P. (1959) 'Adjustment to disability: some observations on patients with multiple sclerosis', *Journal of Chronic Diseases*, 9: 653–70.

Cohen, F. and Lazarus, R. (1973) 'Active coping processes, coping dispositions and recovery from surgery', *Psychosomatic Medicine*, 35: 375–89.

Cooley, C. (1981) 'Self as sentiment and reflection', in Stone, G. and Farberman, H. (eds) *Social Psychology through Symbolic Interaction*, 2nd edn, Wiley, New York.

Corbin, J. and Strauss, A. (1987) 'Accompaniments of chronic illness: changes in body, self, biography and biographical time', in Roth, J. and Conrad, P. (eds) *The Experience and Management of Chronic Illness: Research in the Sociology of Health Care*, Vol. 6, JAI Press, Greenwich, Connecticut.

Cummings, J.H. (1988) 'Salt and water', *Ileostomy Association Journal*, 120: 13–18.

D'Afflitti, J. and Weitz, G. (1977) 'Rehabilitating the stroke patient through patient–family groups', in Moos, R. and Tsu, V. (eds) *Coping with Physical Illness*, Plenum, New York.

Daly, B. and Brooke, B. (1967) 'Ileostomy and the excision of the large intestine for ulcerative colitis', *The Lancet*, 2: 62–4.

Davis, F. (1963) *Passage through Crisis: Polio Victims and Their Families*, Bobbs-Merrill, Indianappolis.

Eardley, A. (1977) 'The sick role and its relevance to doctors and patients', *The Practitioner*, 219: 385–90.

Egbert, L., Battit, G., Welch, C. and Bartlett, M. (1964) 'Reduction of post-operative pain by encouragement and instruction of patients', *The New England Journal of Medicine*, 270: 825–7.

Engel, G. (1968) 'A life setting conducive to illness', *Annals of Internal Medicine*, 69: 293–300.

Fagerhaugh, S. (1973) 'Getting around with emphysema', *American Journal of Nursing*, 73: 94–9.

Field, D. (1974) 'Introduction', in Field, D. (ed.) *Social Psychology for Sociologists*, Nelson, London.

Finan, P. (1988) 'Stomas and appliances', *British Medical Journal*, 296: 1249–1251.

Fussell, K. (1976) 'Common problems of ileostomies and colostomies', *The Practitioner*, 216: 655–60.

Gergen, K. (1971) *The Concept of Self*, Holt, Rinehart & Winston, New York.

Goffman, E. (1968) *Stigma: Notes on the Management of Spoiled Identity*, Penguin, London.

Goffman, E. (1969) *The Presentation of Self in Everyday Life*, Penguin, London.

Goffman, E. (1972) *Encounters: Two Studies in the Sociology of Interaction*, Penguin, London.

Goligher, J., De Domball, F., Watts, J. and Watkinson, G. (1968) *Ulcerative Colitis*, Balliere Tindall & Cassell, London.

Goligher, J., with Duthie, H. and Nixon, H. (1980) *Surgery of the Anus, Rectum and Colon*, 4th edn, Balliere Tindall, London.

Goodman, M. and Sparberg, M. (1978) *Ulcerative Colitis*, Wiley, New York.

Haan, N. (1977) *Coping and Defending: Processes of Self-Environment Organization*, Academic Press, New York.

Hawkey, C. and Hawthorne, A. (1988) 'Medical treatment of ulcerative colitis: scoring the advances', *Gut*, 29: 1298–303.

Hellers, G. (1987) 'Surgery – past, present and future', in Jewell, D. and Mahida, Y. (eds) *Topics in Gastroenterology*, Vol. 15, Blackwell, Oxford.

Helzer, J., Stillings, W., Chammas, S., Norland, C. and Alpers, D. (1982) 'A controlled study of the association between ulcerative colitis and psychiatric diagnosis', *Digestive Diseases and Science*, 27: 513–8.

Herzlich, C. (1973) *Health and Illness: A Social Psychological Analysis*, Academic Press, London.

James, W. (1968) 'Psychology: the briefer course', in Gordon, C. and Gergen, K. (eds) *Self in Social Interaction*, Wiley, New York. Originally published 1892 by Holt, Rinehart & Winston, New York.

Janis, I. (1958) *Psychological Stress*, Wiley, New York.

Janis, I. (1974) 'Vigilance and decision-making in personal crises', in Coelho, G., Hamburg, D. and Adams, J. (eds) *Coping and Adaptation*, Basic Books, New York.

Janis, I. (1985) 'Stress innoculation in health care: theory and research', in Monat, A. and Lazarus, R. (eds) *Stress and Coping: An Anthology*, 2nd edn, Columbia University Press, New York.

Janis, I. and Mann, L. (1977) *Decision Making: A Psychological Analysis of Conflict, Choice and Commitment*, Free Press, New York.

Jewell, D. (1987) 'Factors precipitating relapse', in Jewell, D. and Mahida, Y. (eds) *Topics in Gastroenterology*, Vol. 15, Blackwell, Oxford.

Jones, P.F., Munro, A. and Ewen, S.W.B. (1977) 'Colectomy and ileorectal anastomosis: report on a personal series with a critical review', *British Journal of Surgery*, 14: 615–23.

Keighley, M.R.B., Winslet, M.C., Pringle, W. and Allan, R. (1987) 'The pouch as an alternative to permanent ileostomy', *British Journal of Hospital Medicine*, 286–94.

Kelleher, D. (1988) 'Coming to terms with diabetes: coping strategies and non-compliance', in Anderson, R. and Bury, M. (eds) *Living with Chronic Illness: The Experience of Patients and Their Families*, Unwin Hyman, London.

Kelly, M. (1990) 'Coping with ulcerative colitis and ileostomy: a study of self and identity constructs and their relevance for the coping process', unpublished PhD thesis, in two volumes, Department of Psychiatry, University of Dundee.

Kelly, M. (1991) 'Coping with an ileostomy', *Social Science and Medicine*, 33: 115–25.

Kirkpatrick, J., Thomson, G. and Rogers, A. (1979) 'The quality of life after an ileostomy', *Frontiers of Gastrointestinal Research*, 5: 202–7.

Kirsner, J. (1973) 'Genetic aspects of inflammatory bowel disease', *Clinics in Gastroenterology*, 2: 557–76.

Kock, N.G. (1971) 'Ileostomy without external appliances: a survey of 25 patients provided with intra-abdominal intestinal reservoir', *Annals of Surgery*, 173: 545–50.

Kosa, J. and Robertson, L. (1969) 'The social aspects of health and illness', in Kosa, J., Antonovsky, A. and Zola, I. (eds) *Poverty and Health: A Sociological Analysis*, Harvard University Press, Cambridge, Massachussetts.

Kuhn, M. (1964) 'Major trends in symbolic interaction theory in the past twenty five years', *Sociological Quarterly*, 5: 61–84.

The Lancet (1982) 'Living with an ileostomy', 2: 1079–80.

Langer, E.J. (1983) *The Psychology of Control*, Sage, Beverly Hills.

Langer, E., Janis, I. and Wolfer, J. (1975) 'Reduction of psychological stress in surgical patients', *Journal of Experimental Social Psychology*, 11: 155–65.

Lazarus, R. (1976) *Patterns of Adjustment*, 3rd edn, McGraw Hill, New York.

Lazarus, R. (1980) 'The stress and coping paradigm', in Bond, L. and Rosen, J. (eds) *Competence and Coping During Adulthood*, University Press of New England, Hanover, New Hampshire.

Lazarus, R. and Folkman, S. (1984a) *Stress, Appraisal and Coping*, Springer, New York.

Lazarus, R. and Folkman, S. (1984b) 'Coping and adaptation', in Gentry, W. (ed.) *Handbook of Behavioral Medicine*, Guilford, New York.

Lemert, E. (1967) *Human Deviance: Social Problems and Social Control*, Prentice Hall, New Jersey.

Lennard-Jones, J., Morson, B., Ritchie, J., Shore, D. and Williams, C. (1977) 'Cancer in colitis: assessment of the individual risk by clinical and histological criteria', *Gastroenterology*, 73: 1280–9.

Lewkonia, R. and McConnell, R. (1976) 'Progress report: familial inflammatory bowel disease – heredity or environment', *Gut*, 17: 235–43.

Lindemann, E. (1944) 'Symtomatology and management of acute grief', *American Journal of Psychiatry*, 101: 141–8.

Lipowski, Z. (1969) 'Psychosocial aspects of disease', *Annals of Internal Medicine*, 71: 1197–206.

Lipowski, Z. (1970) 'Physical illness: the individual and the coping process', *Psychiatry in Medicine*, 1: 91–102.

Locker, D. (1983) *Disability and Disadvantage: The Consequence of Chronic Illness*, Tavistock, London.

McCall, G. and Simmons, J. (1966) *Identities and Interactions*, Free Press, New York.

MacDonald, L., Anderson, H. and Bennett, A. (1982) *Cancer Patients in the Community: Outcomes of Care and Quality of Survival in Rectal Cancer*, Department of Clinical Epidemiology and Social Medicine, St George's Hospital Medical School, Report to DHSS.

Mahida, Y.R. (1987) 'Aetiopathogenesis of ulcerative colitis', in Jewell, D. and Mahida, Y. (eds) *Topics in Gastroenterology*, Vol. 15, Blackwell, Oxford.

Mallett, S., Lennard-Jones, J., Bingley, J. and Gillon, E. (1978) 'Colitis', *The Lancet*, 2: 619–21.

Mattson, A. (1977) 'Long-term physical illness in childhood: a challenge to psychosocial adaptation', in Moos, R. and Tsu, V. (eds) *Coping with Physical Illness*, Plenum, New York.

May, D. and Kelly, M. (1982) 'Chancers, pests and poor wee souls: problems of legitimation in psychiatric nursing', *Sociology of Health and Illness*, 4: 279–301.

Mayberry, J. (1985) 'Progress report: some aspects of the epidemiology of ulcerative colitis', *Gut*, 26: 968–74.

Mayberry, J. and Rhodes, J. (1978) 'Aspects of the ileostomy appliance: a survey of the patients' difficulties', *The Practitioner*, 220: 958–61.

Mead, G.H. (1934) *Mind, Self and Society: From the Standpoint of the Social Behaviorist*, University of Chicago Press, Chicago.

Mead, G.H. (1981) 'Self as social object', in Stone, G. and Farberman, H. (eds) *Social Psychology Through Symbolic Interaction*, 2nd edn, Wiley, New York.

Mechanic, D. (1962) 'The concept of illness behavior', *Journal of Chronic Diseases*, 15: 189–94.

Mills, C.W. (1940) 'Situated actions and vocabularies of motive', *American Sociological Review*, 5: 904–13.

Monat, A. and Lazarus, R. (eds) (1985) *Stress and Coping: An Anthology*, Columbia University Press, New York.

Moos, R. and Tsu, V. (eds) (1977) *Coping with Physical Illness*, Plenum, New York.

Morowitz, D. and Kirsner, J. (1981) 'Ileostomy in ulcerative colitis', *American Journal of Surgery*, 141: 370–5.

Morson, B., Dawson, I., with Spriggs, A. (1979) *Gastrointestinal Pathology*, 2nd edn, Blackwell, Oxford.

Moss, C. (1972) *Recovery with Aphasia: The Aftermath of My Stroke*, University of Illinois Press, Urbana, Illinois.

Myers, B., Friedman, S. and Weiner, I. (1977) 'Coping with chronic disability: psychosocial observations on girls with scoliosis', in Moos, R. and Tsu, V. (eds) *Coping with Physical Illness*, Plenum, New York.

Myers, R. and Hightower, F. (1968) 'Critical follow-up of surgically treated ulcerative colitis', *Annals of Surgery*, 167: 920–5.

New, P., Ruscio, A., Priest, R., Petrisi, D. and George, L. (1968) 'The support structure of heart and stroke patients: a study of significant others in patient rehabilitation', *Social Science and Medicine*, 2: 185–200.

Parkes, C.M. (1972) *Bereavement: Studies of Grief in Adult Life*, Tavistock, London.

Parks, A.G. and Nicholls, R.J. (1978) 'Proctocolectomy without ileostomy for ulcerative colitis', *British Medical Journal*, ii: 85–8.

Parsons, T. (1951) *The Social System*, Routledge & Kegan Paul, London.

Pearlin, L. (1985) 'Life strains and psychological distress among adults', in Monat, A. and Lazarus, R. (eds) *Stress and Coping: An Anthology*, Columbia University Press, New York.

Peyrot, M., McMurry, J. and Hedges, R. (1987) 'Living with diabetes: the role of personal and professional knowledge in symptoms and regimen management', in Roth, J. and Conrad, P. (eds) *The Experience and Management of Chronic Illness: Research in the Sociology of Health Care*, Vol. 6, JAI Press, Greenwich, Connecticut.

Pezim, M.E. and Nicholls, R.J. (1985) 'Quality of life after restorative proctocolectomy with pelvic ileal reservoir', *British Journal of Surgery*, 72: 31–3.

Pinder, R. (1988) 'Striking balances: living with Parkinson's disease', in Anderson, R. and Bury, M. (eds) *Living with Chronic Illness: The Experience of Patients and Their Families*, Unwin Hyman, London.

References

Pinder, R. (1990) *The Management of Chronic Illness: Patient and Doctor Perspectives on Parkinson's Disease*, Macmillan, London.

Reif, L. (1973a) 'Beyond medical intervention: strategies for managing life in the face of chronic disease', unpublished mimeo, quoted by Wiener, C. (1975) 'The burden of rheumatoid arthritis: tolerating the uncertainty', *Social Science and Medicine*, 9: 97–104.

Reif, L. (1973b) 'Managing life with a chronic disease', *American Journal of Nursing*, 73: 261–4.

Rideout, B. (1987) 'The patient with an ileostomy: nursing management and patient education', *Nursing Clinics of North America*, 22: 253–62.

Ritchie, J. (1971) 'Ileostomy and excisional surgery for chronic inflammatory disease of the colon', *Gut*, 12: 528–40.

Rosenberg, M. (1981) 'The self-concept: social product and social force', in Rosenberg, M. and Turner, R. (eds) *Social Psychology: Sociological Perspectives*, Basic Books, New York.

Roy, P., Sauer, W., Beahrs, O. and Farrow, G. (1970) 'Experience with ileostomies: evaluation of long-term rehabilitation in 497 patients', *American Journal of Surgery*, 119: 77–86.

Scambler, G. and Hopkins, A. (1986) 'Being epileptic: coming to terms with stigma', *Sociology of Health and Illness*, 8: 26–43.

Schutz, A. (1967) *The Phenomenology of the Social World*, trans. G. Walsh and F. Lehnert, Northwestern University Press, Evanston, Illinois.

Seligman, M. (1975) *Helplessness: On Depression, Development and Death*, Freeman, San Francisco.

Simmons, R., Corey, M., Cowan, L., Keenan, N., Robertson, J. and Levision, H. (1985) 'Emotional adjustments of early adolescents with cystic fibrosis', *Psychosomatic Medicine*, 47: 111–22.

Stoeckle, J., Zola, I. and Davidson, G. (1964) 'The quantity and significance of psychological distress in medical patients: some preliminary observations about the decision to seek medical aid', *Journal of Chronic Diseases*, 17: 959–70.

Stone, G. (1962) 'Appearance and the self', in Rose, A. (ed.) *Human Behavior and Social Process*, Routledge & Kegan Paul, London.

Stone, G. and Farberman, H. (1970) *Social Psychology Through Symbolic Interaction*, Ginn, Waltham, Massachussetts.

Strauss, A., Corbin, J., Fagerhaugh, S., Glazer, B., Maines, D., Suczec, B. and Wiener, C. (1984) *Chronic Illness and the Quality of Life*, 2nd edn, Mosby, St Louis, Missouri.

Stryker, S. (1968) 'Identity salience and role performance: the relevance of symbolic interaction theory for family research', *Journal of Marriage and the Family*, 30: 558–64.

Stryker, S. (1981) 'Symbolic interactionism: theories and variations', in Rosenberg, M. and Turner, R. (eds) *Social Psychology: Sociological Perspectives*, Basic Books, New York.

Tropauer, A., Franz, M.N. and Dilgard, V. (1977) 'Psychological aspects of the care of children with cystic fibrosis', in Moos, R. and Tsu, V. (eds) *Coping with Physical Illness*, Plenum, New York.

Turner, R. (1968) 'The self-conception in social interactions', in Gordon, C.

and Gergen, K. (eds) *The self in social interaction*, Wiley, New York.

Valkamo, E. (1981) 'Ileostomy in ulcerative colitis: a long-term study of the results of conventional (Brooke's) and continent (Kock's) ileostomy in 161 patients', *Annales Chirurgiae et Gynaecologiae*, 70: suppl. 195: 1–81.

Visotsky, H., Hamburg, D., Goss, M. and Lebouits, B. (1961) 'Coping behavior under extreme stress: observations of patients with severe poliomyelitis', *Archives of General Psychiatry*, 5: 423–48.

Walker, K., MacBride, A., and Vachon, M. (1977) 'Social support networks and the crisis of bereavement', *Social Science and Medicine*, 11: 35–41.

Watts, J., De Domball, F. and Goligher, J. (1966) 'Early results of surgery for ulcerative colitis', *British Journal of Surgery*, 53: 1005–14.

Weigart, A., Teitge, J. and Teitge, D. (1986) *Society and Identity: Towards a Sociological Psychology*, Cambridge University Press, Cambridge.

West, P. (1976) 'The physician and the management of childhood epilepsy', in Wadsworth, M. and Robinson, D. (eds) *Studies in Everyday Medical Life*, Martin Robertson, London.

West, P. (1985) 'Becoming disabled: perspectives on the labelling approach', in Gerhardt, U. and Wadsworth, M. (eds) *Stress and Stigma: Explanations and Evidence in the Sociology of Crime and Illness*, Macmillan, London.

White, R., Wright, B. and Dembo, T. (1948) 'Studies in adjustment to visible injuries: evaluation of curiosity by the injured', *Journal of Abnormal and Social Psychology*, 43: 13–28.

Whitehead, W. and Schuster, M. (1985) *Gastrointestinal Disorders: Behavioral and Physiological Basis for Treatment*, Academic Press, Orlando, Florida.

Wiener, C. (1975) 'The burden of rheumatoid arthritis: tolerating the uncertainty', *Social Science and Medicine*, 9: 97–104.

Wilks, S. and Moxon, W. (1875) *Lectures in Pathological Anatomy*, 2nd edn, Churchill, London.

Williams, G. (1984) 'The genesis of chronic illness: narrative reconstruction', *Sociology of Health and Illness*, 6: 175–99.

Williamson, R. and Mortensen, N. (1986) 'Surgical advances in the gut: conservative aggression in the oesophagus, pancreas and colorectum', in Pounder, R. (ed.) *Recent Advances in Gastroenterology*, Vol. 6, Churchill Livingstone, Edinburgh.

Wright, B. (1983) *Physical Disability: A Psychosocial Approach*, 2nd edn, Harper & Row, New York.

Zola, I. (1965) 'Illness behavior of the working class: implications and recommendations', in Shostak, A. and Gomberg, W. (eds) *Blue Colour World: Studies of the American Worker*, Prentice Hall, New Jersey.

Zola, I. (1966) 'Culture and symptoms: an analysis of patients presenting complaints', *American Sociological Review*, 31: 615–30.

Zola, I. (1982) *Missing Pieces: A Chronicle of Living with a Disability*, Temple University Press, Philadelphia, Pennsylvania.

Index